YOUR 'Lose Weight *FAST* the Natural & Healthy-Way DIET',

a simple healthy **weight loss diet** so <u>YOU</u> can live a *better*, *happier*, more *enjoyable* life!

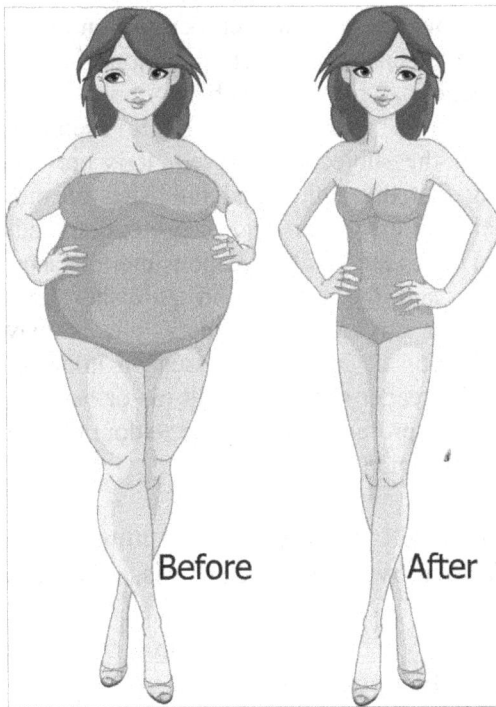

Before   After

By

Wendell & Clarissa Swinton

Published by: Durango Publishing Corp.®
Written by: Wendell & Clarissa Swinton

www.DurangoPublishing.com
Email: books@DurangoPublishing.com

FREE BONUS –

SPECIAL REPORT:

How to *Supercharge* YOUR Metabolism for *Faster* Weight Loss

In this special report you will learn how to burn more calories all day and night with our How to Supercharge YOUR Metabolism for Faster Weight Loss strategies. Using unique and simple to implement ways to supercharge your metabolism you will burn fat and lose weight faster AND keep the extra pounds from making it to your stomach, hips and thighs.

http://www.durangopublishing.com/supercharge-your-metabolism/

**For Your healthier, FASTER weight loss,
Very best regards -**

Wendell & Clarissa Swinton

Forward

As a medical doctor I know that proper eating habits—proper nutrition—are critical to good health. Often that healthy condition is due to reaching and maintaining a proper weight. That's what I found most interesting in "Your 'Lose Weight FAST the Natural & Healthy-Way DIET', a healthy weight loss diet so you can live a better, happier, more enjoyable life!"

Some people seem to eat almost anything and not gain weight. But for most people, following a simple, no-fad, carefully designed diet program is essential. The plans totally detailed in YOUR 'Lose Weight FAST the Natural & Healthy-Way DIET' do just that.

Created for immediate use, this book gives choices that are simple and easy to follow in everyday living. It's not a fad that controls your every movement but an overall program to show you how to make simple choices that result in better, healthier decisions.

Here are just some of the info-packed chapters in Your 'Lose Weight FAST the Natural & Healthy-Way DIET': Portion control, understanding fat, probiotics for balance, measure your body fat, the truth about coffee.

There are also chapters on managing diabetes better, lowering cancer risks, reducing infertility, and eliminating back pain.

Key subjects like stopping depression and increasing energy get excellent coverage to show readers how to cope with these important areas.

This book, written by a knowledgeable team, has a great Index.

YOUR 'Lose Weight *FAST* the Natural & Healthy-Way DIET'

My medical opinion: 5 stars for this great diet book!

Dr. Knox BSc. D.C.
March 2014

For FREE weight loss and dieting tips follow Health, Fitness & Dieting:

on the web: www.DurangoPublishing.com/blog

on Facebook: https://www.facebook.com/pages/Health-Fitness-and-Dieting/1376059622662417?ref=hl

on Google +: https://plus.google.com/u/1/b/103998690891994581249/+Durangopublishing-health-fitness-dieting/posts

on Twitter: https://twitter.com/durangohealth

To receive a FREE copy of our digital newsletter, visit: http://www.durangopublishing.com/tipstricks/

Table of Contents

Section 1

Important Ingredients for Healthy Weight Loss

'Eat less, and burn more'.

These were the words which constantly rang in his ears. He could not continue with his job anymore. For him, everything had finished. The career which he enthusiastically started was about to fade away.

Edward is in his early thirties. With a wife and two small kids, his life was perfect a few years back. However, his life turned upside down when he started gaining weight, and when the doctors classified him as being obese.

For Edward, being obese was not a big deal. With so much passion to make his business grow, he was least concerned about his health. He ignored the words of his nutritionist, who used to constantly remind him to *'eat less, and burn more'*.

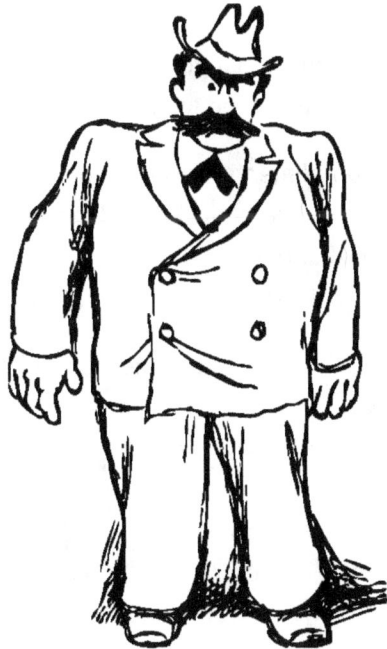

According to the nutritionist, the main cause of Edward's increasing weight was his sedentary lifestyle and regular outings. With money flowing into his house, he never felt the need to dine in. On each weekend, he used to try a different restaurant. When it came to health and food, satisfying the taste buds was Edward's top priority.

He continued searching for new dishes to try on weekends, regardless of how healthy the dishes were.

Lack of physical activity was also an issue in Edward's life. With a lethargic body and a sluggish lifestyle, he never went to the gym to keep fit and active. Being blessed with the latest car, he used to enjoy the car's ride even when he had to go to nearby places.

His business had made him ignorant of his health. The money indeed poured in, but his health was fading away.

Compliments became common in his life when his kids and family members started calling him the best father and the best husband. Little did they know that his life was about to change, and the money was about to vanish.

In short, his ignorance landed him in the hospital three years back when he had a sudden heart attack in the middle of his work. Since then, his health rapidly deteriorated. He could not concentrate on his work, he could not start new projects, and he could no longer manage his business.

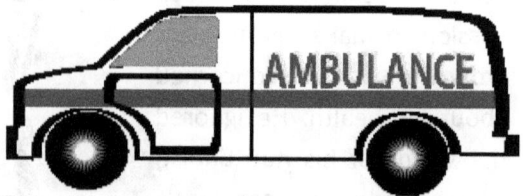

He could not bear the sight of his business going out of his hands. With so much distress creeping in his life, he started falling prey to the world of depression. He regrets not going to the gym, he regrets eating unhealthy foods, and he regrets paying little attention to his health.

This is just one of the many stories you may hear from people who are obese or overweight. Gaining weight is a growing issue in today's world. You will see many people around you who are overweight or obese.

Weight gain affects all aspects of your life. With a fat and lethargic body, you can attract many diseases. There are high chances that your weight gain can make you diabetic. Also, the chances of having serious heart diseases are very high if you are unwilling to reduce your weight.

Weight gain can indeed be discouraging for you. With a bulging body and an inflated belly, you may not feel good about yourself. Inferiority complex often creeps in a person's life when he or she sees slim people around.

We are sure you all love looking smart and healthy. Many men and women reading this book want to reduce their weight, and achieve a trim physique. Many of you want to look like those slim celebrities out there. If you are one of them, then you have landed on the right book.

This book will comprehensively cover all the aspects which you should know to reduce your weight. This book will give you a good idea of how to go about your weight-loss regime.

The information contained in each chapter should not only encourage you to reduce your weight, but should improve your overall lifestyle.

Each chapter is designed to give you the choices which are simple and easy to incorporate in your everyday life. We are not here to give you a strict weight-loss regime which will control your every movement.

Instead, this book will lay down an overall program, providing you with the knowledge to make simple choices that can result in better and healthier decisions regarding your weight.

Starting with the ingredients of healthy weight loss, you will read simple tips which can help you reduce the extra fat you have gained. Then, we will tell you how weight loss will not only bless you with a slim physique, but comes with a lot of additional benefits for your health and life.

All the chapters are stand-alone and can be read in any order that the reader prefers.

While the reasons for weight gain can be many, you need to know that you gain weight when you eat a lot but do not burn off the extra food which you have stored in your body.

This was exactly the reason for Edward's weight gain as well. If you are overweight too, then there are chances that the reason for your weight gain could be similar to the reasons for Edward's weight gain.

Do you know where the unburned food goes to? It gets converted into fat. This fat is then the reason for your weight gain. Hence, if you keep on consuming extra calories, and do not burn them off, you will gain weight. You should therefore follow an active and healthy lifestyle in order to get rid of your extra fat.

As you will see throughout this book, you can reduce your weight if you reduce consumption of certain unhealthy foods, while increasing the consumption of healthy ones. Remember that weight loss is never about starving yourself. The key to reducing weight is to consume healthy foods in a reduced quantity, while burning off the calories gained.

If you do not want to end up with a lifestyle that Edward was following, you need to start planning on reducing your weight. By following the tips given in each chapter, you can be successful in reducing your extra pounds while living a healthier life.

The extra fat around your waist should start to diminish. Your inflated bellies should deflate over time, and you should be able to achieve your desired shape and physique.

The goal of this book is,

> *YOUR 'Lose Weight FAST the Natural & Healthy-Way DIET', a simple healthy weight loss diet so YOU can live a better, happier, more enjoyable life!*

Before adopting any of the suggestions in this publication consulting a physician or health care professional is highly recommended.

Chapter 1 – Portion Control

Now that you know that losing weight is not as hard as you may consider it to be, let us give you some easy tips for reducing the extra calories that you have gained. Ask anyone who has succeeded in reducing weight, and you most likely hear the words 'Portion Control'.

The first thing that may come to one's mind after hearing the words **'Portion Control'** can be the thoughts of starving and skipping your friend's parties. In fact, this is a complete fallacy that to reduce weight, you will have to eliminate certain foods from your diet.

The good news is that you can dine in your favourite restaurant and still control your weight by just controlling the amount of food that you intake. This is what portion control is all about: to understand how much of each food serving is enough for your body, and to control the amount of calories that you intake, while continuing to enjoy the foods that you like.

Let us tell you how portion control helps you reduce weight. An important thing that you need to know about your body is that you gain weight if the number of calories you inject into your body is greater than the number of calories you burn. However, if you practice portion control and reduce the number of calories that you input, your input and output levels will balance. This can result in your weight being reduced.

You should, however, follow an exercise regime to burn additional calories. Portion control decreases the amount of calories that you take in. With reduced input, you will have to do less activity to burn those extra calories. This makes it easier for the body to reduce weight.

Portion control may seem like a daunting task at first, but with patience and practice, it can become one of the biggest reasons for your weight reduction. If you are really serious about reducing your weight, you should learn portion control.

Practicing portion control

There are a number of ways for you to practice portion control. The most important, and easiest, is to learn how to know how much to eat by simply comparing the food size with common everyday objects. There are certain instruments which you can easily use to gauge the right quantity of food to eat.

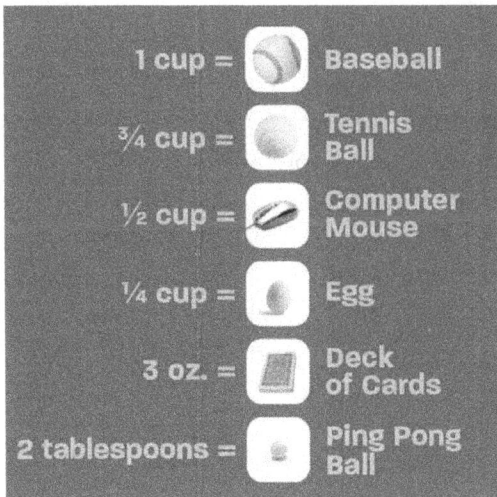

1 cup =		Baseball
¾ cup =		Tennis Ball
½ cup =		Computer Mouse
¼ cup =		Egg
3 oz. =		Deck of Cards
2 tablespoons =		Ping Pong Ball

By this we do not mean that you have to carry a measuring instrument with you every time you eat something. Instead, there are some easy visual aids for you to determine appropriate food servings.

▶ Three ounces of meat, for example, is roughly the size of a deck of cards. It contains 110 calories or one protein serving.

- Same is true for two teaspoons of mayonnaise. It is equal to the size of two quarters, and contains 45 calories, or one fat serving.
- While eating rice, consuming one-third cup, equal to the size of a golf ball, you have around 70 calories.
- Use these, and some more standards to determine the portion sizes and use them the next time you are having a meal, or dining out with family.

In order to reduce weight, you will also have to **sacrifice your appetite** a bit. Eat all that you want to, but in a reduced quantity. We know how appealing a pizza might appear to be, but instead of consuming the whole pizza, consume half of it.

Also, to avoid over eating, make sure you **eat slowly and gradually**. Start talking to your friends or family members while eating. This helps to make you feel full quicker.

If you eat half of your food and still feel hungry, start chewing on something lighter, such as salads. In this way, you will not only consume fewer calories, but you will feel satisfied and full as well. Your appetite will gradually reduce, resulting in your weight being reduced.

Another way to practice portion control and to reduce the calorie intake is to **stay away from meal deals** at restaurants. Your favourite restaurant may be offering the most affordable deal in the town, consisting of all the dishes that you like. But, you should not be tempted to order that deal. These deals will easily ruin your chances of looking slim.

Instead, **consider ordering kids meals** as they will not only satisfy your taste buds, but will also give you less calories to burn. We know it may seem childish for a grown-up to order a kids meal, especially when there is no kid around. But, ignore the weird feelings and eerie eyes and go for this wise option. This is because the happiness you can get once you get slim can be far greater than all the weird feelings

Portion Distortion
What you're served   What's one serving

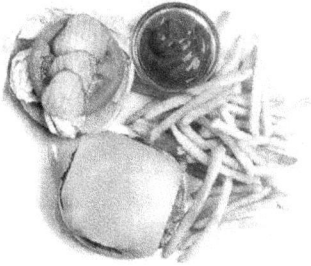

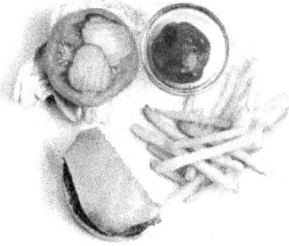

Apart from staying away from meal deals at restaurants, you should also **avoid consuming heavy foods at home**. If you and your family like to eat meat, try cooking meat as a side dish, and vegetables as your main course. In this way you may not only enjoy the taste and nutrients of meat and feel full sooner, but you may also be able to keep those extra calories at bay.

If, however, daily vegetables seem monotonous and boring, tune in to your favourite food channel to experiment with a new vegetable recipe. Eating vegetables can help you significantly reduce weight.

Also**, incorporate vegetable salads** in your daily diet, as salads are a great way to curtail the calories that are harmful for you. They can also help to prevent over eating. Enjoy those green salads with a bit of meat and get fiber and an instant energy boost.

Portion control, however, does not mean that you have to reduce your appetite and diet to a dangerously low level. It also does not mean that you have to starve. You should **never skip meals** if you are planning to reduce weight.

Skipping meals can make you malnourished. It can also increase your temptation to consume certain foods. Hence, it can spoil your chances of getting slim. When you skip a meal, you feel a lot hungrier, pushing you to consume an extra-large portion.

Instead of starving and skipping meals, the best thing to do is to **eat small meals** throughout the day, along with the above portion control techniques. These mini meals can keep your hunger at an even keel and help you keep control of your calorie intake.

Portion control must be present in your weight-loss regime. By practicing portion control, you can feel better and more energetic, and can easily prevent yourself from consuming extra calories. If you want to look like those slim celebrities out there, you will have to practice what those celebrities practiced. That is, you will have to practice portion control.

Chapter 2 – Understanding FAT

What is the first thing that comes to your mind when you hear the word 'Fat'? Is it the enemy which has increased your weight, and which you should avoid? If you are one of those who believe fats to be bad for your weight, then you are partially wrong here.

Just like proteins and carbohydrates, **fat is a source of energy**. Although a certain group of fats can cause weight gain, not all fats are harmful. You should not be scared of them. In fact, some fats are essential for a healthy lifestyle.

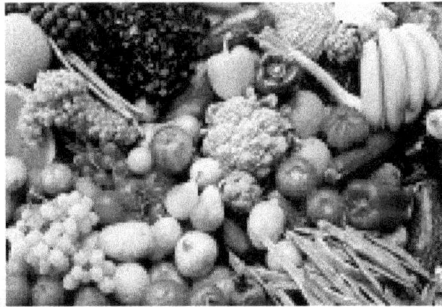

Before we tell you the categories of fats, let us tell you **why fats are vital for your body**.

- ▶ Fat is not just a nutrient for growth and development, it is a source of energy which helps other nutrients to work efficiently in our bodies. It also protects our organs from damage.
- ▶ Fats are also known to stabilize our moods, and to improve our mental health.
- ▶ They act as energy stores in our bodies. This stored fat is then broken down into glucose to supply us with energy, especially in times when there is a shortage in the food supply.

Without some fats, you will not be able to survive. For this reason, the key to reduce weight is not to eliminate all kinds of fats, but to reduce the quantity of certain types of fats which are detrimental for your weight-loss regime.

Let us now tell you the types of fats. There are three major kinds of fats that are found in different foods:

- ▶ Unsaturated fats
- ▶ Saturated fats
- ▶ Trans-fats

These fats can either exist in solid state, or in a liquid state. The fats which are present in a liquid form are known as oils. Some of these fats are important for your survival, while others you should avoid.

Unsaturated fats can be found in the form of oils from plants. These are the fats that are vital for your health, and should be consumed. They still contain high calories; therefore, make sure you eat them in a limited quantity. There are a further two categories of unsaturated fats: polyunsaturated, and monounsaturated.

Monounsaturated fats can be found in certain oils such as olive oil, sunflower oil and peanut oil. These monounsaturated fats may not only reduce the level of 'bad' cholesterol in your body, but can significantly reduce the risk of heart diseases as well. They can help you in reducing your weight, and therefore, you should look for them the next time you go out shopping.

Another kind of saturated fat is **polyunsaturated fat**. This is the fat commonly found in foods such as walnuts, fatty fish, and soybean oil. These polyunsaturated fats also include omega-3 and omega-6 fatty acids, which are beneficial for your health and weight, and should be a part of your daily diet.

Both polyunsaturated fats and monounsaturated fats are the two types of fats which are known as the **'good fats'**. Make them your friends, and include them in your daily diet if you want to reduce your weight and live a healthy life. They still, however, contain a lot of calories. Practice your portion control techniques here and consume these fats in a reduced quantity.

The next two types of fats, which are bad for your health and weight, are **saturated fats and trans-fats**. Saturated fats are usually solids at room temperature, and can be found in foods such as butter, cheese, dairy products, and ice-cream. These are the fats which can be damaging to your health and weight, and should be avoided.

By that we do not want you to completely deprive your taste buds from the taste of ice-cream and cheese. Rather, we want you to consume these fats in a very limited quantity. Also, you should burn these fats away once you satisfy your taste buds.

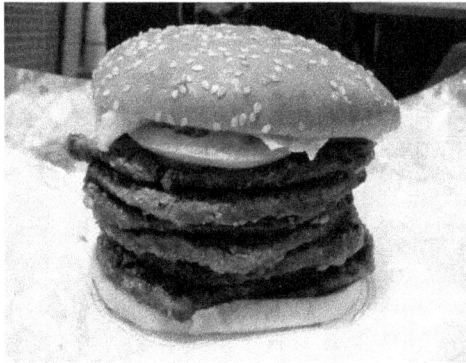

The other partner in crime is the trans-fat. Like saturated fats, it too leads to weight gain. Trans-fat is the manufactured fat, and is made from hardening of vegetable oils. These vegetable oils harden when hydrogen is passed over them.

These fats may be desirable for the manufacturers, but are extremely harmful to your health. You should avoid them, as apart from increasing your weight, they will increase the levels of 'bad' cholesterol in your body, leading you towards different heart diseases.

Consider these 'bad fats' as your enemies and avoid consuming them. Both saturated and trans-fats will increase your calorie intake so much so that you may not be able to burn them off properly. These extra calories can store in your body, leading you to weight gain.

Although fats are known to protect the organs, these bad fats cushion the organs so much that the organs become bulky and heavy, leading to weight gain.

The reason why these fats are harmful for our health is because of their molecular structures. Saturated fats and trans-fats have regular shapes, making it easier for them to stick to our bodies and increase our weights. Unsaturated fats, on the other hand, occur in irregular shapes, and therefore, they cannot stick to our bodies.

So, now that you know what type of fats to avoid, and what type of fats to consume, let us give you some healthy fat consuming tips. You gain weight through fats when you consume saturated and trans-fats, and don't burn them off through exercise. Thus, the key to reduce weight here is to practice a low-fat diet, and to consume unsaturated fats only. Also, exercise regularly, so that you burn what you consume.

Recommended FAT intake

- ▶ According to various nutritionists, your total fat intake should be 20-35% of your calorie intake.
- ▶ Out of this, saturated fats should ideally be less than 10% of your calories.

► On the other hand, say bye to the trans-fats and reduce them to less than 1% of your total calorie intake.

Here is a list of some good fats, which you should consume, and some bad fats, which you should avoid.

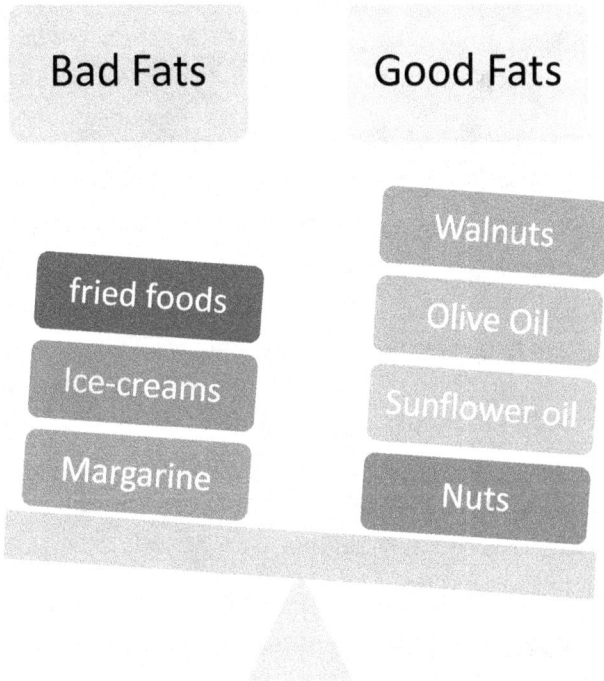

Bad Fats **Good Fats**

Walnuts

fried foods

Olive Oil

Ice-creams

Sunflower oil

Margarine

Nuts

We know how weird it may look if all of your friends are consuming red meat while you are not. But, to get back into shape, you will have to let go of these saturated fats. Instead of having red meat, **try having chicken and fish**. Fish and chicken contain all the 'good fats' which are vital for your health.

Also, **avoid ice creams, whole milk and sour creams**. Try replacing them with frozen yogurt, skim milk and reduced fat ice creams. Instead of using butter and cheese, use vegetable oils. These vegetable oils contain the saturated fats which will keep you in a good shape.

Try reducing the amount of trans-fats to a very low level. **Avoid baked goods, snack foods and solid fats, such as margarines.** No matter how much your friends insist that you eat the cheesy bacon burger, avoid eating fast foods. Also, **check for labels** and buy the products which do not contain hydrogenated oils.

To get the right amount of unsaturated fats which we are constantly talking about, **try cooking with olive oil**. Be creative, and make innovative salads for your meals every day. Also, **consume more avocados and nuts**. You can use them in your dishes and salads as well. All of these foods are rich in unsaturated fats, and should be consumed.

Another very important unsaturated fat to **consume is omega-3 fat**. It will not only help you reduce your weight, but can also increase your mental capabilities. You can consume omega-3 fatty acids by consuming salmon, herring or mackerel. In case you don't like to eat fish, try getting this fat from fish oil.

While walking down the grocery aisle, you will come across a number of appealing food products. Don't look for a 'no-fat' product. Rather, **buy a 'low-fat' product**.

It is a misconception that a 'fat-free' label means that you can satisfy your taste buds without having to worry about your waist and weight. These products may contain low fats, but they will raise your calorie levels through other forms, such as sugars.

When you read the labels of the products, also check the amount of fat included in the packet. If it is a high fat product, it will contain around 17 grams of fat per 100 grams. A low fat product, on the other hand, will have 3 grams of fat per 100 grams. So, make sure you buy a low unsaturated fat product.

The crux of the whole chapter is that unsaturated fats are good for your health, while saturated fats and trans-fats can easily make you bulky. But this does not mean that you completely have to eliminate fats from your diet. You should consume them, but, in a limited quantity. Also, exercise regularly so that you burn those fats away.

By practicing the techniques mentioned above, you will not only gain energy from fats, you will also be able to keep your body in good shape.

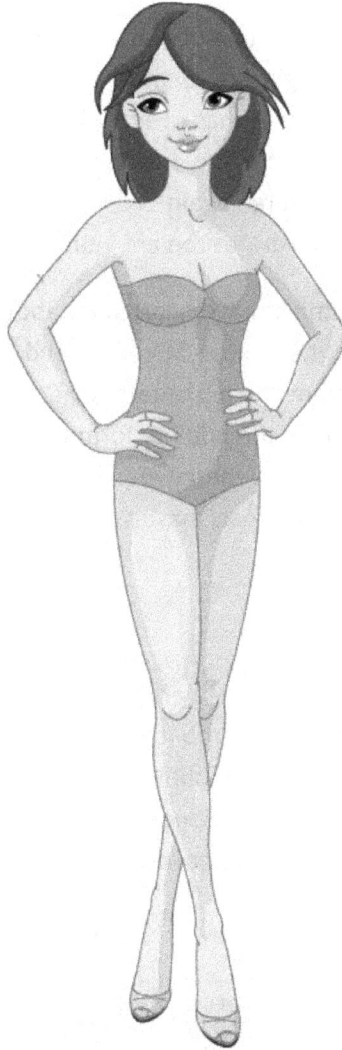

Now let's talk about another important ingredient to manage for weight loss, that is, carbohydrates. Just like fats, you might have heard that carbohydrates are bad for you. You might have been told by several people to follow a low-carbohydrate diet. But, there again you are living under a misconception. Carbohydrates too are vital for your body.

You might have heard a lot about sugars and glucose. Let us tell you the source of sugars and glucose. Carbohydrates are the nutrients that contain sugars. These sugars are then broken down by the body to form glucose, providing you with an ample amount of energy. Carbohydrates can be found in many foods such as cereals, pastas, breads, and anything sweet.

Misconception: A No-carbohydrate diet will help you lose weight.

Remember the very first time you panicked about your weight gain? Most probably, your reaction was to cut down all the sugars and carbohydrates immediately. You probably received advice from friends, telling you to stop eating potatoes, and your favourite pastas as well.

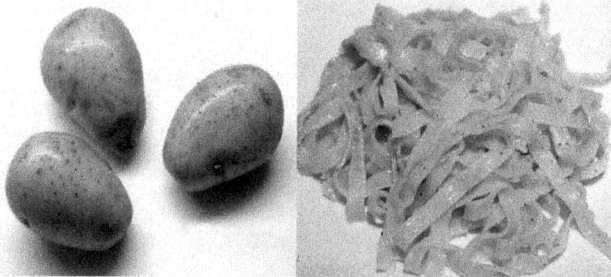

However, if you are one of those who think that a low carbohydrate diet or a no-carbohydrate diet will help you shed those extra pounds, then you are mistaken.

People believe that carbohydrates are the main reason for bulging bellies. In fact, carbohydrates are the essential nutrients which provide energy for your body. They also are important for the brain, as they keep the neurons working perfectly.

We all know that too much of anything will lead you to weight gain. Similarly, just like all the other nutrients, too much of carbohydrates will also increase your weight. But, that does not mean that you should completely eliminate carbohydrates from your diet. In order to keep yourself active and energetic, you will need carbohydrates, but, in a _reduced_ quantity.

Before we go on to tell you why not eating carbohydrates will cause more harm than good, let us tell you some important types of carbohydrates. There are two main types of carbohydrates: simple and complex

Simple Carbohydrates - sugars

Commonly known as 'sugars', these carbohydrates are absorbed faster in the body. You find these carbohydrates in candies, sodas, and fruits, to name a few. Some foods may contain added

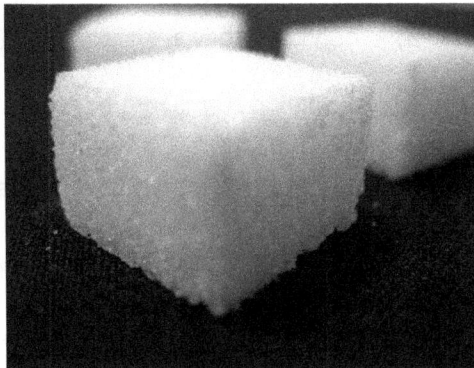

sugars, such as candies and cookies. These are the sugars which are the real culprits. Try to reduce them in your diet.

On the other hand, some foods may contain sugars naturally. These are the foods which are vital for your body, and should not be avoided. Examples of these foods are fresh fruits and milk.

The next time you go out shopping, make sure you read the ingredients, and look for the following culprits:

- Maltose
- Dextrose
- Malt syrup
- Corn syrup

These ingredients indicate that extra sugar is added in the product. So, make sure you do not buy them, as they can cause weight gain.

Complex Carbohydrates – starch and fiber

The second type of carbohydrates is complex carbohydrates. These carbohydrates include starch and fiber. They cannot be used as energy until they are digested.

Starch: You will find starch in foods such as potatoes, white rice, and beans. You might have considered potatoes and rice to be your enemies. But, as you will shortly see, these foods can help you reduce weight.

Fiber: As for fiber, you can get it from foods such as cereals, brown rice and whole wheat bread. These are the nutrients that your body will not digest. However, they are essential for weight loss. Thus, eat foods which contain at least 20% fiber.

Both starch and fiber (let us call them the 'good carbs') should be a part of your daily diet. They can help reduce your weight, and they can also keep your hunger at bay.

Here are some of the reasons why you should be consuming starch, fiber and foods with natural sugars.

- ▶ **They help you lose weight:** It has been proven through research, that a diet containing an adequate amount of the 'good carbs' will help you stay slim.
- ▶ **They increase your satiation:** Fibers and starch have this wonderful property of making you feel full quickly. They have the ability to tell your brain that your body is satisfied now. In this way your hunger is significantly reduced. Thus, you may not crave for more food, leading you to weight loss. Satisfy your taste buds by eating these foods, without worrying about weight gain.
- ▶ **Reduce belly fat:** You may be worried about reducing your bellies. But, here is the good news. Foods containing the good carbohydrates can help reduce your belly fat. These carbohydrates have the ability to burn fats quickly. Your body can lose fat by eating these carbohydrates. Also, they can ensure that the fat is not stored again in the body.
- ▶ **Increase metabolism:** While reducing the fats from your bodies, they preserve your muscle mass. This leads to an increase in metabolism and energy.
- ▶ **Increase your physical endurance:** Do you feel tired and weary quickly after your workout? If yes, then try eating these carbohydrates. They can increase your physical endurance, helping you to exercise and work

more. This can definitely help you in getting a slim physique.

How many carbs to eat daily?

According to various nutritionists, you should consume around 360 grams of carbohydrates. This makes it around 65% of your total calorie intake. Again, make sure not to eat foods with added sugars (*bad carbohydrates*). They are likely to increase your weight.

Some of these **bad carbohydrates** are:

- ▶ Cakes
- ▶ Cookies
- ▶ Sugars
- ▶ Sweetened soft drinks
- ▶ Biscuits
- ▶ Muffins

Examples of healthy carbohydrates

Give your body the energy boost that it needs to reduce those extra pounds by consuming the following foods:

Foods	Nutrition	Additional information
Potatoes	100 grams = 77 calories 100 grams = 2.2 dietary fiber 100 grams = 17 carbs	You might have been surprised to see potatoes on this list. Potatoes are not only rich in starch; they have high vitamin contents as well. Therefore, try potatoes in your salads and enjoy its weight reducing

		benefits.
Barley	½ cup = 97 calories ½ cup = 3 grams dietary fiber ½ cup = 22 carbs	Just like potatoes, barley too is rich in starch. It has the ability to curb down your hunger, making you feel full.
Whole wheat pasta	½ cup = 195 calories ½ cup = 1.7 grams fiber ½ cup = 39 carbs	Ignore all those who have been telling you to avoid pastas. Pasta too has the ability to reduce your hunger. Consume up to ½ cup of pasta daily.
Strawberries	100 grams = 33 calories 100 grams = 2 grams fiber 100 grams = 8 carbs	Strawberries are full of natural sugars and fiber. They can give you instant energy and a helping hand in weight reduction. If you are tired of not having anything sweet lately, try strawberries.
Whole wheat bread	2 slices = 160 calories 2 slices = 8 grams fiber 2 slices = 30	Consume 100% whole wheat bread to help you reduce weight.

	carbs	
Beans	½ cup = 109 calories ½ cup = 8 grams fiber ½ cup = 20 carbs	They are full of fiber and can help you reduce your waistline. Make sure you use canned beans with little sodium.
Green peas	½ cup = 67 calories ½ cup = 4.5 grams fiber ½ cup = 12.5 carbs	Just like all the foods mentioned above, peas can reduce your hunger. They have the ability to tell your brain that you have had enough. Thus, your hunger, and eventually weight can be reduced. Also, it can provide some other important nutrients as well.

These are some of the foods which should be a part of your daily diet. A very important reminder here is not to go on a low-carbohydrate diet. Instead of keeping the carbohydrate level up to 65%, some people reduce it to less than 30%. It will have a number of disadvantages for your body.

Firstly, it will not make you slim. You will be under a lot of stress once you cut down on your favourite carbohydrate foods. This can lead to a boost in your appetite. Eventually you will probably have more food. Thus, your chances of getting slim will reduce with a low-carbohydrate diet.

Secondly, it increases your stress. You may shout at your children as you may be low in energy. You may be fighting with your boss. This is all because of a low-carbohydrate diet. It lowers your energy so much that you feel sad and irritable.

Thirdly, it can increase your cravings and your bellies. With fewer carbohydrates in your body, you can suffer from constipation. Constipation then leads to your bellies getting swelled up.

If you want to achieve your dream of getting a slim physique, eat up to 65% carbohydrates. Don't go for a low-carbohydrate diet. It can easily ruin your chances of getting slim.

Chapter 4 – Power of Proteins

You probably have heard a lot about the importance of proteins for your bodies. We are here to inform you of the importance of proteins for weight loss. Just like carbohydrates, proteins too ensure weight loss.

Proteins are the nutrients found in foods such as eggs and meat. They are demanded by all parts of the body. Be it the bones, or the brains, they all need proteins for their development. It has the ability to protect your body from different diseases as well.

But most importantly, proteins have the power to reduce your bellies. They are known to increase your metabolism, and to curb down your hunger. If you want to look slim, then you should definitely have a protein rich diet.

Let us tell you the reasons why proteins should be a part of your diet.

Proteins help you burn fats and calories

Perhaps the primary concern of every man and woman reading this book will be to burn fats and calories. But, here is the good news: include proteins and carbohydrates in your diet, and see those extra fats burning down.

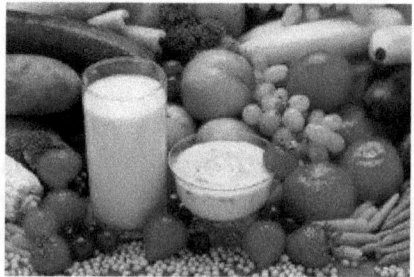

By consuming a protein-rich diet, you can get slim at a faster rate.

Protein curbs down your hunger

You may have been concerned about your stomach feeling hungry all the time. You might have been irritated about your body not feeling full. Well, here we have a remedy for your problem. Eat a protein rich diet, and see your hunger being reduced. A protein-rich diet has the power to make you feel satisfied and full for a longer period of time.

You may then not crave for more food. This can ensure that your daily calorie level is under control, helping you to maintain your weight.

Protein increases your metabolism

We all know that exercise is essential for weight loss. However, when you exercise and control your diet, your muscle mass starts to reduce. Your metabolism level drops down and you feel lethargic all the time. In order to avoid this miserable feeling, try a protein-rich diet.

Proteins can ensure that you do not lose muscle mass during weight loss. Also, proteins provide energy to your liver, which in turn increases your metabolism. You will not feel lethargic and weary all the time. Proteins can ensure that your metabolism level is increased up to 30%.

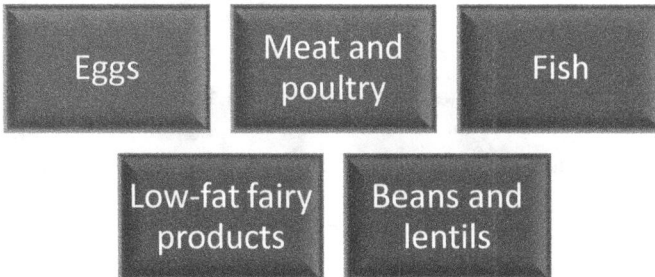

Eggs	Meat and poultry	Fish
Low-fat fairy products	Beans and lentils	

Inspired by proteins? Let us tell you some of the sources from which you can gain those proteins:

Recommended Protein Intake

Now that you know how important proteins are to your bodies, let us look at how much you are supposed to eat. You should keep in mind that in order to get the above weight-loss benefits of proteins, you need an adequate amount in your diet.

In order to lose your weight, nutritionists recommend that your total calorie intake should contain at least 30% proteins. That means that if you are consuming a 2000 calorie diet, then you need up 150 grams of protein daily.

In case you cannot figure out how much calories your protein foods contain, remember that **1 gram of protein has 4 calories.** The process is quite simple. Just multiply the grams by 4 to figure out the number of calories. For example, for 150 grams of proteins, you consume 600 calories (150 x 4 = 600).

Also, before filling your dishes with proteins, make sure you include the right type of protein. Some of these proteins are obtained from animals. Examples of these proteins include meat, bacon and dairy. When these animal proteins are processed, they contain some saturated fats as well. These saturated fats are harmful for your weight. Try avoiding processed meat such as bacon, ham, and sausages.

The next time you cook or order anything, remember the following:

- ▶ 1 cup cooked rice contains 4 grams of proteins (16 calories)

- 100 grams meat or chicken will have around 25 grams of proteins (100 calories)
- 200 grams yogurt contains 10 grams of proteins (40 calories)
- ½ cup soybeans will provide you with 8.5 grams of proteins (34 calories)
- 40 grams of cheese will have 10 grams of proteins (40 calories)

Using this information, choose your daily protein intake wisely. Also, make sure you increase proteins in your breakfast.

Consuming proteins in breakfast can boost the weight-loss benefits of proteins. You can, for example, eat an omelette and drink a smoothie with proteins. You should, however, make sure that your breakfast is low in saturated fats.

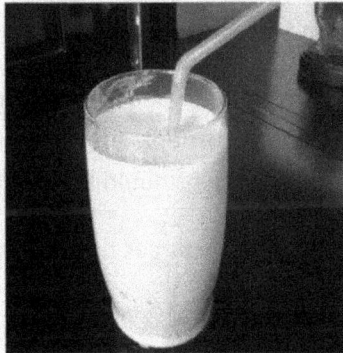

We know that this information might have made you excited to eat more proteins from now on. But, beware; eating too many proteins can actually jeopardize your health.

Some foods which contain proteins may also contain saturated fats. Thus, eating too many proteins can cause high consumption of saturated fats. These saturated fats are the enemies of your slim physique, and can cause weight gain.

Also, eating more proteins and fewer carbohydrates means low fiber intake. Low fiber intake can cause constipation and swelling of your bellies.

High proteins can also damage your kidneys. This can then lead to loss of calcium and other important nutrients. Therefore, make sure you take the recommended amount of proteins only. Do not over consume proteins, as they can have the opposite effect.

Complete and incomplete proteins

Proteins are made up of amino acids which are vital for your body. Not all proteins will provide you with these essential amino acids.

All those amino acids which will provide you with all the necessary nutrients are called **Complete Proteins**. These are the proteins which should be incorporated into your diet.

Some of the sources of these complete proteins are:

- ▶ Fish
- ▶ Eggs
- ▶ Milk
- ▶ Yogurt
- ▶ Meat

While all types of proteins should be included in your diet, there are some which will not provide you with all the essential protein nutrients. They are called **Incomplete Proteins**. They should be combined with other nutrients, so that you experience the true power of proteins.

Some of the sources from where you can get these proteins are:

- ▶ Nuts
- ▶ Beans
- ▶ Corns
- ▶ Peas
- ▶ Grains

Try eating these foods by combining them with some other sources of proteins. For example, include beans in your salads, along with peanuts, to get all the nutrients. Try eating grains in combination with some dairy products. Or, be a little creative and enjoy sesame and flax seeds with some yogurt.

Moreover, you should eat all those proteins which are low in fats. These proteins are called **Lean Proteins**. They can help you reduce your weight quickly, by letting your stomach feel full for a longer period of time. Below is a list of some healthy lean proteins for you to eat:

Healthy Protein Sources

Eggs	Eggs are the most economical source of proteins. Available cheaply everywhere, eggs are rich in proteins and low in fats. Open up the creative part of your mind, and try different dishes with eggs, especially for breakfast.
Fish	Fish is not just good in taste; it is also high in proteins. Try salmons and other cold water fishes. They will have low fats, and can give you the benefits of weight-loss.
Chicken and	

poultry	Yes, you can get the taste of your favourite chicken recipes without having to worry about weight gain. These poultry dishes are rich in proteins. Just make sure that you remove the skin before eating.
Beef	People believe that reducing weight means reducing beef. This is not true. Beef is a good source of proteins and other nutrients. Just make sure you remove any fat that you see around the raw beef.
Beans and peas	Are you a vegetarian? If yes, then you should increase your consumption of beans, lentils and peas. These foods will provide you with ample amount of proteins, and can reduce your weight. You can try different recipes of beans and peas in salads.
Low fat dairy products	Low fat dairy products are not just low in fats; they are rich in proteins as well. You can add them in different recipes to get a good taste and a healthy weight loss.

Breakfast is the best way to start your protein-rich day. Eat eggs, yogurt, skim milk and oatmeal in your breakfast. For a peppery start, try a little bit of chicken or sausages as well.

After a good protein-start, fill up your day with a protein rich lunch as well. You can try fish, turkey sandwiches and crunchy vegetables. Also, fill up your salads with beans and lentils to get a protein boost.

After a tiring day at home, or at work, you need an energy filled dinner. For this you need to fill your dinner with carbohydrates and proteins. You can safely have a meal containing fish, chicken or turkey. Just be sure to practice portion control, and to eat a limited quantity.

You can also fill your protein quota by eating snacks and deserts throughout the day. Again, make sure you do not consume over and above the recommended amount of calories. Also, after all of these meals, make sure you burn these calories away as well.

Have a protein rich diet and enjoy your physique coming back to your desired shape.

Chapter 5 – Fruits for Fitness

Have you ever wondered why those celebrities have flawless skins and bodies? That is because they consume fruits. If you are serious about losing your weight, and keeping yourself in shape, then start eating fruits. Fruits can bless your bodies with a perfect shape.

While exercising and cutting down on calories, you lose energy. You need nutrients to replace those energies with something which is not high in calories. Fruits are those sources of energies: they are the nutrients which can help in weight loss and provide you with an ample amount of energy.

Why should fruits be a part of your daily diet?

▶ **Fruits are low in calories and fat**
  For a successful weight-loss diet, you need foods with low calories and fats. Fruits usually do not contain any 'bad fats'. Also, they are low in calories, and are ideal for people who are concerned about their weights.

▶ **They are rich in fiber**
  Fiber is one of the most important ingredients for weight reduction. It helps you curb down your hunger, making you feel full sooner. Fortunately, you can get doses of fiber cheaply by consuming fruits daily.

▶ **They contain antioxidants**
  Fruits also contain antioxidants which helps us keep ourselves in good shape. Antioxidants also lower the blood pressures and can fight back many diseases. Accordingly, you should eat fruits daily so that your body feels good.

▶ **Fruits are rich in nutrients**

Fruits will not only aid in reducing your weight, they will provide you with some essential nutrients as well. These nutrients will ensure that your body has an adequate amount of energy to perform different chores. Also, they will keep you hydrated.

For that reason, instead of joining a slimming centre, try being friends with these fruits. They can give you all that you need for a healthy weight loss.

But, how many fruits should you eat daily?

The amount of fruits to eat daily depends on your gender, age and daily workout regime. Nutritionists suggest that you should consume a **minimum 5 fruits and vegetables daily**. In terms of serving, this is equivalent to **2 cups of fruits daily**.

Here are some of the fruits that are equivalent to one cup. Each cup of fruit will give you approximately 65 calories. **2 cups of fruits will give you an average of 130 calories**.

1 small apple

½ cup dried fruits

1 orange, peach, pear or grapefruit

1 cup

8-10 large berries, cherries or grapes

1 slice of melon or pineapple

1 large banana

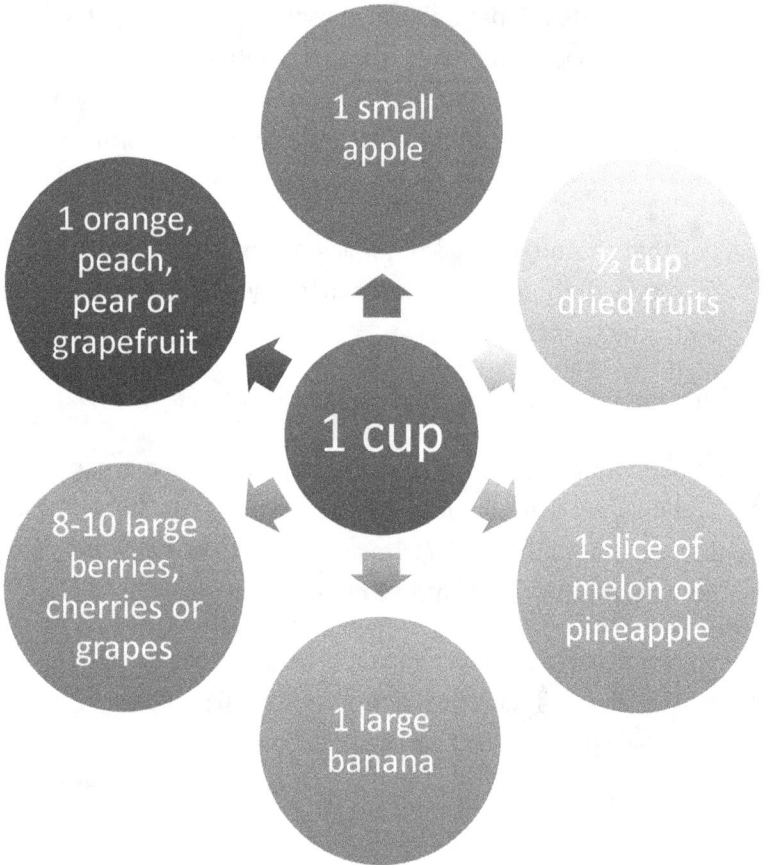

Now that you know how many fruits you have to eat daily, let us tell you the fruits to eat.

Berries

Berries such as strawberries, raspberries and blueberries are an excellent source of essential nutrients. They are low in fats and calories, and high in fiber. The fiber in these berries will help you feel satiated, keeping your hunger at an even keel. One cup of strawberries, for example, will give you around 50 calories and 3 grams of fiber.

As compared to other fruits, these berries are also low in sugars, and will therefore not lead to weight gain. Blueberries also have the power to keep you active throughout the day. There is no reason left for you to say no to these lovely berries. Try having their juices early in the morning to see your weight being reduced in a few days.

Grapefruit

Grapefruit is also considered as an important fruit for weight loss. Although it is a bit sour in taste, this fruit can help you lose weight quickly. Grapefruit contains few calories. 1 cup of grapefruit will provide you with 74 calories. Also, they have high water content. This high amount of water is useful for making you feel full.

While giving you some weight loss benefits, grapefruit can also lower your cholesterol. It is also helpful in preventing some forms of cancer. Grapefruits should be a part of your daily fruit intake. If you do not like the fruit because of its sour taste, try drinking its juice with some salt. It will not only taste good, but can help you reduce weight in a few weeks.

Watermelon

Watermelon is known for its high water content. Just like grapefruit, this high water content is beneficial for weight loss. It will signal your brain that you have had enough, making you

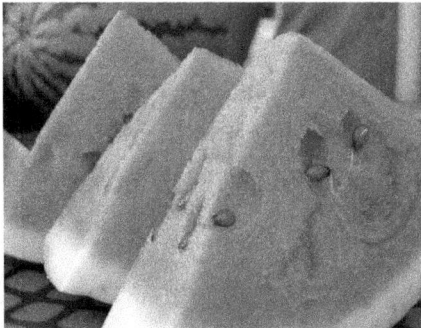

feel satiated early. Moreover, it will help you digest several foods.

Watermelons are also rich in fibers. This fiber rich food again will help you curb down your hunger. Thus, you have here a not-so-expensive fruit to help you shed those few extra pounds.

Apples

After a tiring day at the gym, you definitely need some energy boosters. Apples are one of those energy boosters which you should eat.

Apples are a great source of energy, and can keep you active throughout the day. They are also rich in other vitamins and minerals. This is helpful as when following a weight loss regime, you need extra nutrients to prevent you from being malnourished.

It also contains small amounts of sodium, which is an added benefit. They are also rich in antioxidants and low in calories and fats. As the old saying goes,

"Eat an apple a day, to keep those extra pounds away."

Avocado

Avocados have a bad reputation when it comes to healthy fruits for weight-loss. This is because they have a relatively higher fat content as compared to other fruits. However, the fat inside avocados is the 'good fat' and should be consumed for weight loss.

Avocados are known to increase the metabolism rate, and can help in reducing excess fat from your body. They also contain omega-9 fatty acids, which are healthy for your bodies.

Bananas

If you want to lose your weight by eating healthy foods, then bananas should be a part of your daily fruit intake. Bananas are rich in carbohydrates and a little rich in calories too. You need not worry here though, as these calories are fat-free calories.

Wondering why, despite being a little high in calories, bananas are still in this list? This is because bananas are rich in carbohydrates and fibers. These are the nutrients which will help you feel satiated for a longer period of time. Furthermore, bananas are a great source of energy. Therefore, go bananas, and try eating bananas in your breakfast.

This list includes many other fruits as well, which will have all the weight-loss benefits. Some of these fruits are papaya, peaches, oranges and mangoes. Consume these fruits as well to get your bellies in a good shape.

An important reminder

If we have told you that fruits will help you in reducing your weight, this does not mean that you should eat as many fruits as you want to. Limit your fruit intake to a maximum of 2 cups only. This is because if you fill your quota of calories through fruits only, you may get unnecessary amount of sugars in your body as well. This increase in your sugar level can then become a reason for your weight gain.

Thus, just like any other food, limit your intake of fruits to enjoy its weight-loss benefits. Here we have some healthy fruit recipes for you.

breakfast	lunch	dinner	Snacks
•Smoothie •Pure fresh juice	•Fruits in salads	•Fruit salad as a dessert	•Eat fruits instead of oily snacks

Breakfast

▶ You can have a fruit smoothie at breakfast for an energetic start.
▶ Also, instead of a smoothie, drink a glass of 100% pure juice. Make sure no extra sugars are added to it.

Lunch

▶ Lunch is the time where your energy starts draining. Refill this energy by including fruits in your lunch meals.
▶ You can have fruits by adding them in your salads.
▶ Try different recipes such as mango roll-ups, apple apricot salad and apple raisin salad.

Dinner

▶ Make your dinners interesting and healthy by including fruits in your meals.
▶ Make a fruit salad and enjoy this as a delicious dessert.

You also have to ensure that you eat a healthy meal even when you are dining out. No matter how stupid it may seem, you should order something with fruits in it. Here again, make sure the recipe has low calories and low 'bad fats'.

Fruits are vital for your weight-loss regime, as they can reduce your hunger, increase your energy level, and reduce weight quickly. Consume the recommended amount of fruits daily so that you can quickly achieve your dream of looking like those celebrities.

Chapter 6 – Vegetables for Variety

Do you remember your grandma who used to constantly force you to eat vegetables? You might make a lot of weird faces at the sight of those vegetables. But, you should listen to your grandma's advice if you haven't already.

Start loving vegetables and make them your best friends.

We are saying this because vegetables have the power to reduce your weight, and give you a perfect shape. They will also fill you up with all the essential nutrients which you have been missing out on.

They don't have a good reputation when it comes to tasty foods. However, you will find vegetables on the plates of all those who are serious about reducing their weight.

Still not convinced about giving up meat for boring vegetables? Read these few pointers. They will tell you how essential vegetables are for your body.

They help reduce your hunger.

▶ Try eating 5-6 plain crackers, and you will see that your hunger is not reduced. Now, on some other day, eat 6 cups of sliced cucumbers. Feeling more satisfied? This is the beauty of vegetables. They can make you feel full, while giving you less calories.

Those crackers and cucumbers will give you the same calories, but cucumbers can make you feel full. Switch to vegetables and reduce your hunger.

They are powerful antioxidants.

▶ Just like fruits, vegetables too contain antioxidants. These antioxidants are helpful to reduce your extra pounds. They also protect you from various diseases. Get your hands on vegetables and protect yourself from diseases and fats.

They are rich in fibers.

▶ We have been constantly talking about the benefits of fiber for your body and weight. These vegetables too are a great source of obtaining fibers. Fibers will not only help you in reducing your weight, they will also aid in absorbing other nutrients.
These fibers will also act as energy boosters. So, you will not feel dull at the end of the day if you eat vegetables daily.

Vegetables are your cheap and sincere friends who will assist you in weight-loss. These low calorie foods will not only give you energy and essential nutrients, they will also help you in burning your excess fat. They come with a lot of varieties, so you don't have to worry about a monotonous diet. Try eating vegetables daily to get the most out of them.

Just like fruits, the amount of vegetables to eat varies according to your age, gender and daily routine. For simplicity, **remember that:**

> You should eat a minimum of 5 fruits and vegetables daily

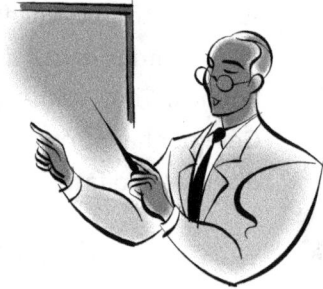

This is equivalent to **2 cups of vegetables daily.** We have a simple chart for you to remember how much of vegetables will be equal to 1 cup:

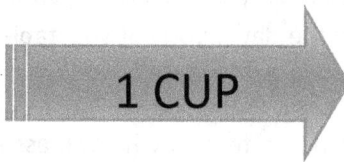

1 CUP →

- ► 2 medium carrots
- ► 1 large baked potato
- ► 1 ear of corn
- ► 5-6 broccoli florets
- ► 11 inches long celery

Now that you know how many vegetables you should eat, let us give you an overview of the varieties of vegetables available. Grocery stores can leave you confused with the number of choices available. Choose vegetables from these options to get back into shape.

Spinach

Spinach is a great vegetable for you to eat. It is high in fiber and will therefore be a great tool to reduce weight. It is also high in all the nutrients which a diet should include. Examples of these nutrients are vitamins, calcium and magnesium. There are a number of ways for you to eat spinach. One popular way is to eat spinach in your salads.

Broccoli

Your mother might have run after you to force you to eat broccoli when you were a kid. The reason why you were pressured to eat it was because it is a great source of all the essential nutrients. Just like spinach, it is rich in vitamins, calcium and magnesium.

Also, you will be happy to know that it contains no fats. You should definitely include it in your diet as it will not be harmful for you. It will provide you with carbohydrates and proteins too, and both of them are needed by your bodies to lose weight.

Kale

Low in calories and high in other nutrients, this vegetable is a great source to reduce weight. Change your taste a bit and use kale in your soups. These soups will satisfy you early, and will reduce your hunger. Hence, your weight will be under better control.

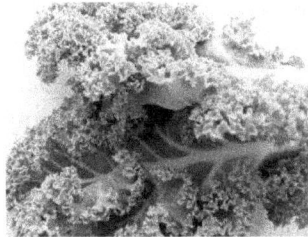

Cabbage

Cabbages are also popular in weight-reducing diets, as they are low in calories. These cabbages are rich in fiber, and can thus have a slimming effect. You can eat cabbages in a variety of ways. You can cook or steam them. Or, use them in your salads to make them tasty.

Mustard greens

Tired of the usual vegetables and meats? Try this tasty vegetable to

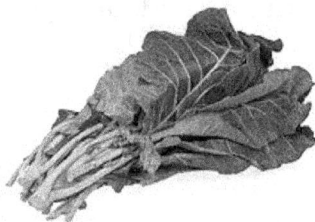

53

experience a slimming effect. They are low in calories and rich in proteins.

Swiss chard

This is another vegetable which should be a part of your daily diet. It is also low in calories, as one serving of Swiss chard contains just 7 calories. You can eat this chard with butter beans to give a different taste to your taste buds.

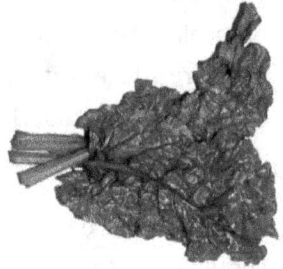

Potatoes too can cause weight loss.

We are pretty sure you have been strictly told to exclude potatoes from your diets. This is, in fact, a misconception that to reduce weight you have to sacrifice your liking for potatoes.

The reason why potatoes have a bad reputation here is because people use potatoes with high-calorie foods. Of course you are not supposed to eat French fries every time you are with your friends. But, one or two potatoes in your daily salads wouldn't reduce your chances of getting slim.

Potatoes are actually rich in carbohydrates, rich in proteins and low in calories. You already know how much proteins and carbohydrates are useful for your bodies. Eat potatoes, in a limited quantity, to get the benefits of these nutrients.

Potatoes also have the ability to eliminate some of the problems with your digestive systems. They will also detoxify your body and help prevent wrinkles. Do not deprive your taste buds from the taste of potatoes, and use them daily.

You should however, not eat a lot of potatoes. Also remember to not eat potatoes with fattening foods and oils. This can have an opposite effect on your weight.

Besides the vegetables mentioned above, there are many other vegetables which will have the same effect. Before choosing to cook any vegetable, just be sure that it is low in calories.

Still confused about how to eat vegetables? Here are some of the ways through which you can easily diversify your vegetable meals.

Make soups

Ward off the chilly weather with some tasty hot soups. Make them with some crunchy vegetables and enjoy a meal full of nutrients.

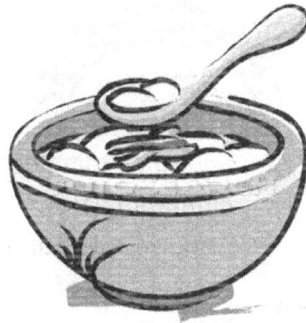

Eat them raw

Fill in your calorie quota by munching crunchy raw carrots or cool cucumbers. Raw vegetables will be the most beneficial for you. There are many vegetables which can be eaten raw. Choose from the variety of options available and get a slim physique.

Go Italian

We are sure you love pastas and pizzas. Give your taste buds a treat and fill your pastas and pizzas with vegetables to get a healthy meal.

Disguise them in different dishes

You can also hide your favourite vegetables in different dishes to get a different taste. Include vegetables in your lasagna and Indian dishes to enjoy the benefits of weight-loss. Just be sure to not consume more bad fats and calories.

Use them with sauces

Enhance the flavours of your favourite vegetables by dipping them into various sauces. This will not only make your meals a bit different, but will also fill you up with nutrients.

It can be boring to eat vegetables daily. But with the above options and some extra meal tips, you can learn to love vegetables.

Breakfast

- ▶ Add some tomatoes and onions to your omelettes, for a different taste.
- ▶ Also, you can drink vegetable juices in the morning. Drink a glass of carrot juice to not only get healthy skin, but to get a good physique as well.
- ▶ Use spinach or avocados with your early morning sandwiches.

Lunch

- ▶ Have those flavoursome dishes of meat or chicken with vegetables in them.
- ▶ Also, fill your salads up with green vegetables.

Snacks

- ▶ You can use celery stalks with cheese, or olives with cheese.

- Make a small chicken sandwich with lettuce and cheese on it.
- You can also have a variety of salads as snacks. Tune into your favourite food channel to look up some tasty recipes for salads.

Dinner

- Dinner is the time when you should try to have vegetables, so that you get all the energy back which has been drained out of you.
- If you're having pizzas or pastas, let your children top them up with their favourite vegetables.
- You can also eat steak with a healthy salad and some mashed potatoes.
- You can also top your turkey and chicken recipes with different vegetables.

We hope we have convinced you to listen to what your grandma used to say when you were a kid. If you want to be in perfect shape, then these vegetables are a must. Eat them daily to reduce the extra fat in your body.

Chapter 7 – Nuts and Seeds for Nutrition

Are you tired of eating the same old vegetable and fruit salads as snacks? Do you want to give yourself a break and try something different and healthy? If yes, then switch to nuts and seeds.

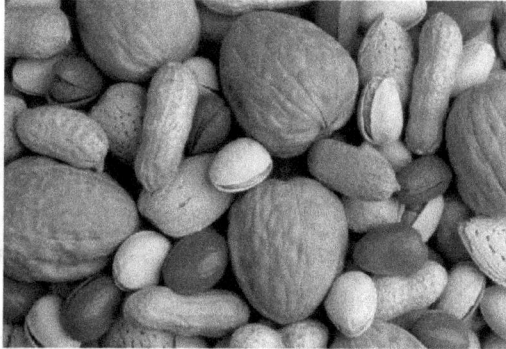

Nuts and seeds are known for their high nutrition and health benefits. Nature has blessed us with a huge variety of nuts and seeds to choose from. These nuts and seeds can help you reduce your weight, while giving you all the essential nutrients that your body needs.

You might have heard that nuts and seeds are high in fats, and should not be consumed. People are right when they say that some nuts and seeds have high fat contents. However, what they probably don't know is that these fats are unsaturated fats, which are vital for your weight-loss regime.

Nuts and seeds are not new in town. People have been consuming them because of their nutritional benefits since ancient times. You might also have seen your grandparents munching a handful of nuts.

With your busy schedule, and an already tough diet regime, you might not be consuming enough nuts these days. Here are some of the benefits of nuts to convince you to start eating them.

They help reduce your hunger

We have been constantly telling you about all those foods which can make you feel less hungry. Well, here is another addition to that list. Nuts and seeds are also famous for reducing your appetite.

They can make you feel full in a short time, hence reducing your cravings for more food. So, the next time you feel hungry and have already had enough calories, try munching a handful of nuts and seeds. They can magically let your hunger die.

They are rich in fiber and proteins

Many nuts and seeds are loaded with fiber and proteins. By now, you should be aware of the importance of fiber and proteins for your weight-loss regime. Get your hands on these nuts and seeds to fill up with fibers and proteins.

High in essential nutrients

For a healthy weight loss, you know that you need some extra nutrients as well. Fortunately, nuts and seeds are rich in all those nutrients. They contain magnesium, zinc and minerals. These nutrients are essential for your body, but are not normally consumed in a proper amount.

They are also rich in certain antioxidants, such as vitamin E. These antioxidants are needed by your bodies during weight-loss. Eat these nuts and seeds, and fill your bodies with all these essential nutrients, without worrying about high calorie levels.

59

High in unsaturated fats

Unsaturated fats are nothing to get scared about. They are, in fact, needed by your bodies for healthy weight reductions. You can also fill your quota of unsaturated fats by eating nuts and seeds daily.

Nuts and seeds are rich in poly and monounsaturated fats, which are vital for your bodies. They are also rich in omega-3 fatty acids. These fats can also help protect you from various diseases.

Prevention from diseases

The nutrients inside nuts and seeds can help protect you from major diseases, such as cancer. Risk of getting cancer can decrease if you eat nuts and seeds daily. This is the reason why people who have cancer are advised to include nuts and seeds in their diets.

The fatty acids in these nuts and seeds can also help in maintaining your cholesterol levels. This, in turn, reduces your risk of heart diseases. So, eat nuts and seeds daily and prevent yourselves from weight gain and dangerous diseases.

> ## Eat 1 serving of nuts and seeds daily.
>
> ## Where 1 serving = 1 oz.

What is the amount of nuts and seeds to eat daily?

Check the list below.

One oz. of nuts and seeds is equivalent to:

▶ 14 halves of walnuts
▶ 24 almonds
▶ 28 peanuts
▶ ¼ cup sunflower seeds
▶ 18 cashews
▶ 47 pistachios
▶ 1 tablespoons of flax meal
▶ 6 Brazil nuts

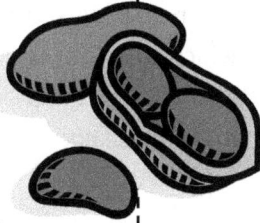

So far, you know that nuts and seeds will give you all the essential nutrients, and that you should eat 1 serving of them daily. But, with so many options available at the grocery stores, choices can be a bit difficult to make.

Let us help you with this. Here we have for you some of the healthiest nuts and seeds. These are the ones which you should definitely buy the next time you go shopping.

Almonds

Almonds are one of the healthiest nuts to go for. Rich in protein and vitamins, these nuts can help you lose weight quickly. Eating almonds daily will also provide you with some healthy unsaturated fats.

So, the next time you make a sweet dish or some snack, ask your children to decorate the dishes with some almonds. You just have to make sure that your children don't put in all the almonds. Almonds have to be eaten in limited quantity, since too many almonds can increase your calorie intake.

Walnuts

Walnuts are also included in the list of healthy nuts, since they are rich in unsaturated fats. They also contain omega-3 fats, which are vital for your weight-loss. Eating walnuts daily can also fill you up with some essential nutrients, such as manganese and copper.

Peanuts

Peanuts are a good source of healthy unsaturated fats too. They also contain vitamin E and magnesium, which can help your body to maintain a good shape.

You also have the option of peanut butter here. Peanut butters are low in carbohydrates, and can safely be consumed by those who have diabetes. You can use 2 tablespoons of peanut butter daily in your breakfasts for a healthy start.

Pistachio nuts

Feeling hungry after lunch? Try eating some pistachios, and see your hunger being reduced. Pistachios are also famous for being rich in unsaturated fats.

You should, however, not consume more than 1 ounce of pistachios. This is because pistachios are relatively high in calories, and should be consumed in a limited quantity.

Cashews

Cashews too are rich in unsaturated fats. They are also a good source of antioxidants and zinc, both of which are needed by our bodies.

There are many other nuts which will give you the benefits mentioned above. Some of those nuts are butternuts, hazelnuts, and pine nuts. You can safely use 1 serving of these nuts as well to experience a healthy weight loss.

Now that we have talked a lot about nuts, let's turn towards seeds. In order to have a healthy and nutritious diet, you should definitely get your hands on the following seeds.

Chia Seeds

If you ever search for the benefits of chia seeds, you will have an endless list in front of you. Chia seeds are one of the healthiest seeds to eat as they are loaded with all that your body needs.

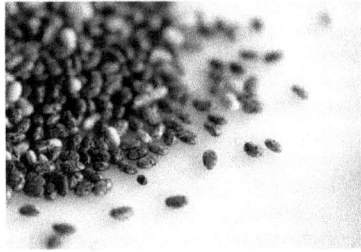

They are filled with proteins, fibers and fatty acids, all of which are helpful for weight loss. They can also fill you up with energy if you eat them after a tiring day. However, remember that **you should eat no more than 1 tablespoon of chia seeds daily**. Eating chia seeds daily can also help you prevent a few diseases.

Facts about Chia Seeds

- ► Contain 10 times more fiber than rice.
- ► Have 6 times more calcium than milk.
- ► Have 8 times more omega-3 fatty acids than salmons.
- ► Will give you 2.5 times more proteins than beans.

Thus, buy chia seeds as soon as you can, and start eating them daily for a healthy diet.

1 serving = 1 tbsp.

Pomegranate seeds

Pomegranate seeds are also important for weight-loss. These low-calorie foods are rich in fiber and antioxidants. These seeds will also fill you up with some essential nutrients, such as vitamin C and potassium.

Before eating pomegranate seeds, remember that:

1 serving = ½ cup.

Hemp seeds

Another healthy seed is the hemp seed. It is believed to be one of the richest sources of unsaturated fats. Hemp seeds are also rich in protein, so they can provide you with a healthy diet.

1 serving = 1 tbsp.

Sunflower seeds, sesame seeds, flax seeds, and pumpkin seeds

These seeds are also included in the list of healthy seeds. All of them are rich in proteins, fibers and unsaturated fats. Thus, including them in your daily diet will not only help make you healthy, it can also keep your weight under control.

Before eating these seeds, make sure you know their serving sizes.

- ▶ **Flax seeds**: 1 serving = 1 - 2 tbsp.
- ▶ **Pumpkin seeds**: 1 serving = ½ cup.

▶ **Sesame seeds:** 1 serving = ¼ cup.
▶ **Sunflower seeds:** 1 serving = ¼ cup.

We hope you will buy bags of these nuts and seeds the next time you go out shopping. With a huge range of options to choose from, choose raw nuts and seeds over roasted and salted ones.

Roasting and processing nuts can destroy some of their essential nutrients, so they will be of less use to you. Also, avoid sugar coated nuts, since they can be high in calories.

Before buying nuts, you should also make sure the nuts look clean and healthy. Unclean nuts often contain harmful bacteria.

Although eating them raw is the best option to go for, here we have some tips to give your taste buds a different taste. You can use your favourite nuts and seeds in the following foods:

▶ Rice
▶ Pasta
▶ Soups
▶ Breakfast cereals
▶ Salads

Now that we have given you so much information about nuts and seeds, rush to your favourite store now and grab bags of your favourite nuts and seeds. After you come back, pour them out in a bowl, switch on your favourite television show, throw yourself in a comfortable sofa, and enjoy a healthy treat.

Chapter 8 – Probiotics for Balance

Imagine yourself eating bacteria to reduce your weight. We are sure the thought is scary. But, believe it or not, it has been proven through research that bacteria can help you lose your weight.

You should, however, not get scared at the thought of eating bacteria. This is because the bacteria that we are talking about here are the friendly bacteria. These small healthy bacteria, known as **probiotics**, are microorganisms that help prevent a lot of diseases.

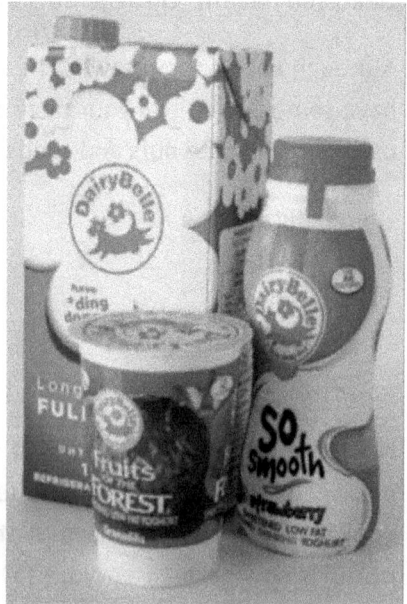

It is true that we take antibiotics to fight against harmful bacteria when we are ill. But, the bacteria which we will be talking about here are the ones which go along well with our bodies. They are often found naturally in foods, such as yogurt.

They are not just well-known for helping you treat certain illnesses; they are now also famous for reducing your weight. Therefore, if you wish to lose some belly fat, try taking probiotics. Here are some of the **benefits of adding probiotics in your diet**.

It will help you improve your digestive system

Probiotics can be very useful if you are experiencing certain digestive problems. Antibiotics are often proscribed to fight against harmful bacteria. But, while they remove harmful bacteria, these antibiotics remove a small quantity of friendly bacteria as well, leading to an imbalance in the digestive system.

These were the friendly bacteria which were helping out your system to maintain good health. When these friendly bacteria are removed, an imbalance is created in your bodies, and you experience certain problems.

You may start experiencing diarrhea, which can make it difficult for you to continue your weight-loss regime. We are sure you do not want to spoil your hard work of maintaining your health by falling ill for a few days.

In this case, it is necessary for you to eat something which can help you remove these illnesses. Taking foods containing probiotics is a remedy here. This is because **probiotics have the power to cure diarrhea up to 60%.**

It can restore the imbalance of friendly and bad bacteria, and can improve your health. In this way, you can be physically and mentally ready to focus on your task, which is weight loss.

Diarrhea is not the only thing which can jeopardize your health, and weight-loss regime. You may also experience irritable bowel movements. These irritable bowel movements can often lead to cramps, pain and constipation.

It would be hard to follow your diet while suffering from an upset stomach, and severe cramps. Thus, it is necessary here for you to take foods with probiotics.

Help prevent urinary problems

Eating small quantities of foods containing probiotics can save you from a few urinary problems as well. Just like in the digestive system, probiotics can help maintain the balance in the urinary system. In this way, you may not experience any urinary problems, helping you to concentrate on weight loss.

They will help maintain a woman's health

For all you women reading this chapter, if you are a sufferer of bacterial vaginitis or yeast infections, read on. These two diseases are caused by an imbalance in woman's bodies, and can cause major discomforts for women.

They may also stop you from working out, or following a weight-loss regime. Therefore, it is advisable for you to eat foods with probiotics, so that the balance of good and bad bacteria is maintained in your body. It is only when the balance will be maintained that you will be able to lose your body fat.

Eat foods with probiotics for a healthy immune system

Do you want to save yourself from diseases? If yes, then eat foods with probiotics. Probiotics have the power to improve your immune system.

Without a healthy immune system, you can be exposed to various diseases, which can hinder your weight-loss regime. It is advised that you should eat foods with probiotics, so that you do not catch diseases easily.

They can help you reduce your weight

You may not know this, but if you are obese, then your intestinal flora will be different from that of normal people. High consumption of fat and low consumption of fiber is probably a reason for this difference.

This is because high consumption of fat can lead to an imbalance of bacteria. This can then become a reason for weight gain. Probiotics, however, have the power to burn the excess fat. They can also restore the balance of friendly and bad bacteria. When everything will be back to normal, you can start losing weight.

We are not making statements out of thin air. It is in fact **proven by research**. Researchers conducted a study, in which they took 125 obese men and women. They were then divided into two groups, where each group was supposed to follow a weight-loss diet for 12 weeks. They then had to maintain their weight for another 12 weeks.

For the first 12 week period, one group was given probiotic pills, while the other group was given a placebo. After the first 12 weeks were over, it was observed that women who were given probiotics pills reduced 9.7 lbs (4.4 kg) of their weight.

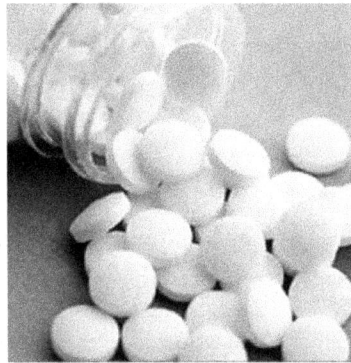

The placebo group, on the other hand, lost around 5.5 lbs (2.5 kg) only. Women in the probiotics group were able to reduce more weight because **taking probiotics had accelerated weight-loss**.

After the initial 12-week plan, these groups had to maintain their lost weight for another 12-week. After this phase was over, it was observed that each women in the probiotics group reduced weight up to 11.7 lbs (5.3 kg). The placebo group, on the other hand, was unable to reduce further weight.

Thus, we have two very important findings from this study:

- ▶ Women who take probiotics will lose more weight as compared to those who don't.
- ▶ Women who take probiotics will be able to maintain a healthy weight, even after completion of a probiotics-rich diet.

These two findings should be enough to convince you to incorporate probiotics in your daily diets. They can help you gain a smart physique in a short span of time.

You must have noticed that we have only revealed the effect of probiotics on women. Well, here we have some sad news for men. The research described above has only shown positive results with women. Men were not affected by a probiotics-rich diet.

Reasons for this are still unknown. The researchers, however, are trying to find out the causes. So, you should not get disheartened completely.

Foods containing probiotics

Do you want to make your bellies happy? If yes, then try these foods and increase your chances of a healthy weight loss.

Yogurt

Yogurt is perhaps the most convenient source of probiotics. Easily available in almost all the grocery stores, yogurt will supply a good amount of friendly bacteria to your bodies.

This yummy yogurt can also cure diarrhea and irritable bowel movements. Yogurt is a great source of weight reduction, as it helps in burning excess fat.

Yogurt is also a rich source of vitamins and essential nutrients. 1 serving of yogurt can easily fill you up with the necessary amounts of zinc, potassium, vitamin B5 and vitamin B12.

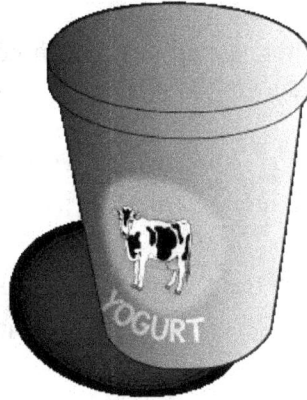

Therefore, eat **8-10 ounces of yogurt daily** and get loaded with essential nutrients and friendly probiotics. You should, however, not be tempted to buy yogurt just by looking at its fancy packaging. Always look for the label **"live, active cultures"** before buying yogurt.

This is because some of the yogurts you buy are pasteurized. Since pasteurization reduces the benefits of yogurt, it will not help as much to lose weight. Only pick those yogurts which contain active bacteria.

Milk

Yes, milk can also fill you up with some friendly bacteria. When going out to buy milk, look for the label of "acidophilus milk". This is the type of milk which has been fermented with bacteria, and will be beneficial for your health, and weight loss regime.

71

Use limited amount of acidophilus milk though, as it can also increase your calorie levels.

Sour pickles

Some of the sour pickles you eat also contain friendly bacteria. Thus, eating pickles can help keep some digestive problems at bay.

You should, however, buy naturally fermented pickles. Also, look for pickles in which vinegar is not used. This is because these pickles will befit you the most.

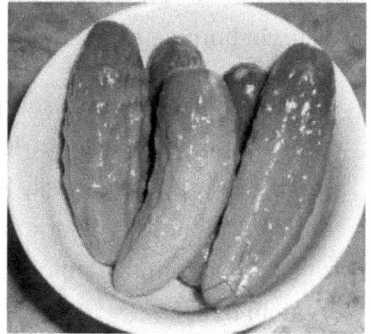

Supplements

Probiotics are not just found in fermented foods, they can also be obtained through probiotic supplements, such as capsules, liquids and powders. Although they will not provide you with extra nutrients, they are rich sources of friendly bacteria.

You should, however, use these supplements as per your doctor's advice. This is because some of the brands can be of low quality, and thus, dangerous for your health.

Some recommended foods with probiotics

Here are some unpasteurized foods, which will supply you with ample amount of friendly bacteria.

- ► Plain yogurt
- ► Pickles
- ► Kefir

- ▶ Tempeh
- ▶ Miso
- ▶ Kombucha Tea
- ▶ Kimchi

Daily dosage for these probiotics is not yet set. However, doctors recommend that we should consume food which would provide us with around 1-10 billion live organisms. It may sound too much for you right now, but in terms of capsules, it is equivalent to 1-2 capsules of probiotic supplements daily.

To conclude, bacteria are not always harmful for us, as there are some bacteria which can actually aid in weight loss. Concentrate on weight loss while maintaining a healthy body by consuming probiotics daily.

Chapter 9 – Ditch the Salt

Do you like to add more salt to your dishes? If yes, then you need to stop, as you might hinder your chances of losing weight. Here in this chapter, we will be telling you the relationship between consumption of salt and gaining weight.

Recommended amount of salt by food agencies is 6g per day, but many people over look it and consume about 10-12g of salt each day. This can not only cause you disappointment in weight loss, but can also land you in blood pressure problems, which is a major cause of strokes and heart attacks.

We know how tasteless your dinner and lunch can be without salt. But, what is more important for you? Is it maintaining a good taste, or is it losing weight? We are sure it is losing weight. In order to achieve your dream of looking like slim celebrities, you need to cut down your consumption of salt.

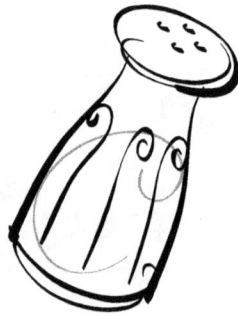

Salt and sodium

Before we go on to tell how harmful salt is for your bodies, we want to clear a misconception. People think that it is the consumption of salt which can be harmful. It is, however, wrong.

It is the consumption of sodium which can be problematic for you. Sodium is a mineral which is needed by our bodies to maintain fluid balances, and to control nerve impulses.

Too much sodium, however, can be dangerous for our health. Since table salt contains 40% sodium, it too can be dangerous for us if over consumed.

Let us now see why salt can be your enemy, and why you should not add more salt to your dishes.

Salt can increase your weight

Directly, salt doesn't cause your body to gain weight. You may be surprised to know that there are no calories in salt.

If this is the case, then how come salt leads to weight gain?

It is in fact the high consumption of salt which can lead to weight gain. With the recommended consumption of salt, the sodium level in your body is balanced. But, as you increase salt consumption, the levels of sodium in your body can rise.

Sodium has the power to attract water. As soon as the level of sodium in our bodies gets high, we feel a lot thirstier. Have you ever wondered why eating so many peanuts can trigger your thirst mechanism? This is because peanuts can increase the amount of salt in your bodies, causing you to drink more water.

Because of high levels of sodium, you may then rush to drink more water. This has a serious disadvantage, as our bodies can temporarily retain water until the sodium levels are balanced. This retention of water can lead to swelled tummies. It can eventually lead to you gaining some extra pounds.

The extra water added to our bodies is also carried away to our skins, through blood. This causes our skins to swell up, and we get a bloated look. Avoid consuming high salt, as it can make you look puffy and blown up.

Salt can increase your blood pressure

Since sodium has the power to hold water, high levels of sodium can increase the level of water in our bodies. This attraction of water can make it difficult for our kidneys to remove excess water. The extra water puts pressure on our blood vessels.

The added pressure is dangerous for our hearts, as it leads to high blood pressure. Blood pressure is further increased when our arteries grow stronger and thicker to cope with the extra strain. This increase in the blood pressure can be so dangerous that it can lead to bursting of some arteries.

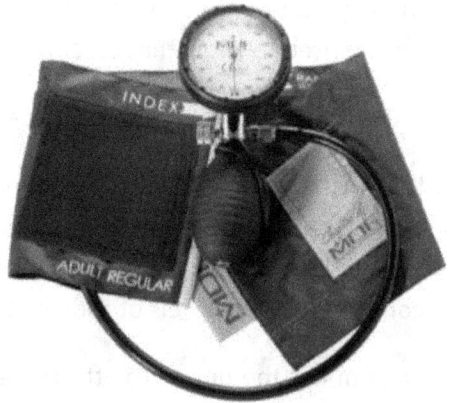

When the arteries leading to the heart get clogged, our heart's ability to pump blood will decrease. An increase in the consumption of salt can lead to a chain reaction, in which all parts of the body can be affected.

Salt and pressure on kidneys

Also, as the level of water is increased, the pressure on kidneys increases too. Our kidneys become ineffective in removing excess water from our bodies. This extra water puts strain on our kidneys, leading to potential kidney damage.

Reduce your consumption of salt, so that extra water does no harm to your body.

Restriction of sodium – A bad practice

You might be wondering if the solution is to reduce your consumption of salt by a great amount. You might think that by restricting salt in your diet, the excess water may decrease.

If you reduce your consumption of sodium below the recommended level, your body can temporarily reduce the excess water. You might be able to lose around 3 pounds in a few days if you consume around 1,000 milligrams of sodium.

You should, however, note that the happiness you can get may be temporary. 1,000 milligrams of sodium is a very low quantity of sodium to consume. Over time, a low quantity of sodium can lead you to several other diseases and imbalances.

Therefore, you should not **restrict** your consumption of sodium too much if you want to stay healthy. You should in fact, **lower** your sodium intake.

Restricting water intake – A bad practice

Some of you might be thinking to restrict water intake to reduce your bloated bellies. This, however, is a very dangerous practice, and should not be carried out.

Water is essential for almost all parts of our bodies. Restricting your water intake can do more harm than good. It can negatively affect all the organs which use water for their functioning.

I make sure that I do not add more salt to my meals, so why do I get bloated then?

This is a common concern of many women. The key to reduce weight here is not just to limit your intake of salt through meals at home. You may not know this, but the foods you eat when you dine out are more dangerous for you than the table salt you use at home. They contain high amounts of sodium. Thus, concentrate on reducing your intake of processed foods as well.

Also, restricting water can have no effect on weight-loss. It can rather aggravate the problem, and damage our organs. Therefore, the key here again is neither to restrict water or sodium. You should just **lower** your consumption of salt in general, and sodium in particular.

It may be interesting to note that 75% of sodium comes from processed foods. 15% of sodium is added through salt in the meals we cook, while less than 10% comes from fruits and vegetables. Since a larger proportion of sodium comes from processed foods, it is necessary for us to reduce their consumption.

Tips for reducing salt through processed foods

Here are some of the processed foods which can be dangerous for your health, if over consumed.

- ► Frozen dinners
- ► Food in brine
- ► Pizza
- ► Sauces

- ▶ Breakfast cereals
- ▶ Canned soups

We are not asking you to completely ban these foods from your lives. Some of these foods, in fact, are good for your health. However, you should just practice portion control here, and consume them in a limited amount.

Also, look for low sodium products the next time you go out shopping. You should also look at the labels of the products, and see whether the amount of sodium is high or low.

Remember that you should ONLY consume 6g of salt daily.

Reducing salt intake at the dinner table

Here are some of the tips for reducing salt intake when cooking meals at home:

- ▶ Use ingredients with low levels of sodium.
- ▶ You can cook rice and pasta without using salt.
- ▶ Switch on your favourite food channel and look for low salt recipes.
- ▶ You can also buy a low salt cookbook.
- ▶ While cooking chicken, use ginger, oregano, rosemary or sage. This will add taste to your foods, while reducing the amount of salt needed.
- ▶ Cook your favourite dishes of meat using bay leaves, onion, pepper or sage to reduce salt addition.
- ▶ While cooking potatoes, use oregano, parsley, onion and ginger to reduce salt consumption.

You can use this tip to remember your daily salt intake.

1 pinch of salt = 1 gram of salt

Reducing salt when eating out

- ▶ Order meals with low-sodium ingredients.
- ▶ If possible, ask the chef to cook your meals with low salt.
- ▶ Also, avoid taking cheese with your salads. Salads made at some restaurants can already contain a high amount of salt. Adding cheese to it can increase your sodium levels.

Use these tips to make sure that you eat a lower amount of sodium when dining out. We know it may seem weird to request the chef to cook your food with low salt. But, your health and weight are at stake here. Nothing should be embarrassing and weird for you when it comes to weight-loss.

Reducing salt when buying fruits, vegetables and meat

Some fruits and vegetables also contain high amounts of salt. To reduce your salt intake through fruits and vegetables, make sure you use fresh fruits, instead of canned ones. Canned ones can have relatively high salt contents.

Same is true for poultry and meat. Buy fresh meat and poultry, instead of canned ones. You should also limit your intake of processed and smoked beef.

By following the tips mentioned above, you may be able to prevent yourself from having a puffy figure. Also, follow these tips to come back to your normal physique, if sodium has already blown you up.

We know how upset your taste buds can get once you decide to reduce your salt intake. Nothing may taste flavoursome to you without salt. The first few days can especially be difficult.

However, you need not worry here as your taste buds will soon adjust to low-salt flavours. It may take around 3 months for your taste buds to fully adjust to the new taste. Every dish will become tasty then, even with less salt in it.

Reduce your consumption of salt to prevent yourself from a bloated figure. Try practicing the tips mentioned above, to get back to your dream physique.

Chapter 10 – Dump the Sugar

Do you love candies and cakes? We are sure you will reply in the affirmative. Well, here in this chapter, we will be asking you to make certain sacrifices. If you wish to reduce your weight, then you need to cut down your sugar intake.

You need to restrict your intake of candies and cakes, no matter how much they appeal to you. This is because sugar can be a very powerful tool to jeopardize your weight. Instead of weight loss, it can lead to weight gain. Therefore, it is beneficial for you to give up your sugar intake.

Sugar facts:

► It will be helpful to note that **1 gram of sugar contains 4 calories.**
► Therefore, if you consume 1 teaspoon of sugar, you will take in 16 calories.

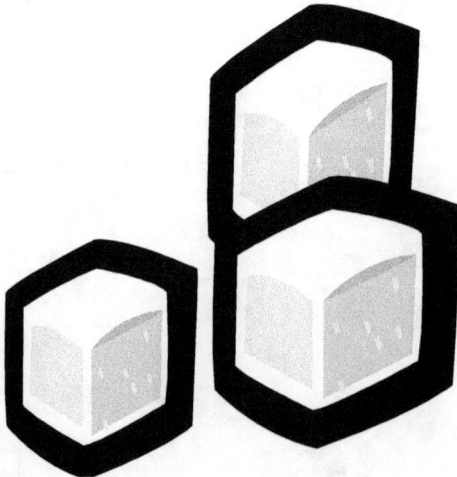

Natural and Added Sugars

There are two kinds of sugars which can be found in many foods: natural and artificially added. **Natural Sugar is the good sugar you should look for**. It is naturally present in fruits, vegetables, beans and nuts.

These sugars will be beneficial for your health and will provide you with extra nutrients. These will not harm our weight-loss regimes, as they are present in small quantities in foods. They just sweeten up our foods, without creating problems for our weight. Give your taste buds a sweet taste by consuming safe fruits and vegetables.

Added sugars on the other hand are artificially added to sweeten a food. **Added sugars are the bad sugars which you should avoid**. Manufacturers usually add extra sugar to sweeten a dish, to preserve a product or to ferment it. You will easily see these bad sugars in all the candies and cookies. These sugars can jeopardize your chances of looking slim, and hence, should be avoided.

Added sugars can increase your weight

Added sugars are good for nothing. They will no doubt enhance the flavour of your dishes. They can also satisfy your sweet tooth. But, they can fill you up with extra calories.

Natural sugars also contain calories, but they provide us with essential nutrients as well. A strawberry, for example, is not just sweet in taste; it is also rich in vitamins and fiber. Added sugars, on the other hand, will just add calories to your diet, without providing you with anything healthy.

By consuming more candies, cakes and ice-creams, you will just increase your calorie intake and add excess fat to your body. This can quickly increase in your weight within a few days.

Also, if you love sugars, you might be replacing good sugars with bad sugars. You might be eating more candies instead of vegetables. This is wrong, as apart from increasing your calories, you are missing out on all the essential nutrients of fruits and vegetables.

If you want to reduce your weight, the last thing you need is added sugar.

Can increase fat in your liver

Added sugars contain fructose in them. When we eat candies, the fructose in it goes to the liver where it is metabolized. If you eat a lot of candies, a large amount of fructose can gather in our livers.

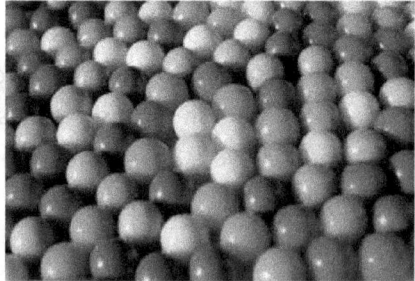

Now, if you exercise enough and burn off the fructose, then you need not worry here. But, in case you do not do that, the excess fructose in your body will convert into fat. This can not only lead to an increase in your weight, it can also lead to many liver problems as well.

This is because the fat stuck on our livers can hinder its functioning. Reduce your consumption of bad sugars to give your liver some peace.

Can lead to diabetes

When you consume too many candies and cookies regularly, the sugar level in your blood can significantly rise. This can result in the pancreas releasing insulin to remove excess sugar from your blood.

However, if you are constantly eating sugars, your pancreas will be regularly releasing insulin to remove excess sugar. Eventually, there can come a time when your pancreas may stop responding, and cannot release insulin.

At that point in time, you can become a diabetic patient. Therefore, you should avoid creating stress for your pancreas by restricting your sugar intake.

Can accelerate aging process

We are sure all the people reading this chapter want to look slim and younger. Well, for that to happen, you will have to restrict your intake of bad sugars.

If you regularly eat extra sugars, your body can stop releasing human growth hormone. This is the hormone which is responsible for making you look young. Allow your bodies to release this hormone, and look a few years younger, by limiting sugar intake.

Can destroy your immune system

Bad sugars also have the disadvantage of paralyzing your immune system temporarily for a few hours. However, if you constantly eat foods with these bad sugars, your immune system is likely to get permanently damaged. You should avoid sugars to protect yourself from diseases.

Some other reasons why you should give up your favourite candies:

- ▶ They can cause anxiety and depression
- ▶ Can lead to hyperactivity
- ▶ Can cause food allergies
- ▶ Can lead to an imbalance of mineral in our bodies
- ▶ Can reduce the absorption of magnesium and calcium in our bodies

Here are some of the foods which you need to minimize in your diets. In this way, you can be protected from the harmful effects of sugars.

Avoid carbonated drinks

Carbonated drinks should never be on your list of drinks to buy. This is because they contain, on average, 15 teaspoons of sugar. This means that they will fill you up with approximately 240 calories, with no nutrition at all.

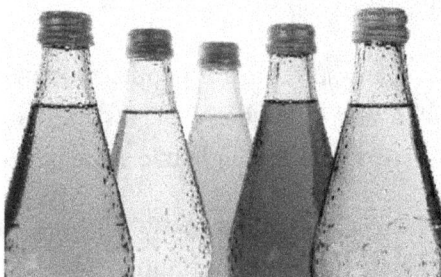

Also, don't go for diet sodas, as they contain some harmful sugars. These sugars will not only increase your weight, but can also jeopardize your health.

Avoid cookies, candies, desserts and ice-creams

Although these candies and ice-creams come in fancy packages, you should not be tempted to eat them. This is because they contain high amount of calories. 100 grams of cookies and candies, for example, will fill you up with more than 50 grams of sugar.

Ice-cream too is harmful; as one ice-cream bar will provide you with 17 teaspoons of sugar. These foods also contain trans-fat, a bad fat which significantly increases your weight.

Avoid fruit juices

When fruits are converted into juices, a large amount of water and fiber is removed from them. Water and fiber can help you feel full sooner. This is how you are saved from over consuming sugars when you eat fresh fruits.

However, when fiber and water are removed from the fruit, you do not feel satiated quickly. This can lead to more consumption of fruit juices in general, and sugars in particular.

Your level of calories can therefore rise, and you can gain weight. This is the reason why a juice made out of 2 oranges can never make you feel full, while eating 2 oranges can do so.

> ## Daily recommended level of sugar
>
> You should not eat more than 24 grams of sugar daily.
>
> Note that 24 grams = 6 teaspoons = 100 calories

Now that you have a fairly good idea about the foods to avoid, let us help you with avoiding these foods by providing you with some tips.

Breakfast

Make your breakfasts healthy and sugar free, by avoiding all types of jams and marmalades. Also, do not eat a cereal if 100 grams of it contains more than 3 grams sugar. You should also not eat yogurts if some sort of sweetener has been added in it.

In order to reduce your sugar intake, you can eat porridges and unflavoured shredded wheat. You can also have eggs, bacon and sausages in the breakfast if you want to avoid sugars. Just make sure that the sauces you use do not contain added sugars.

Snacks

You should not destroy your chances of looking slim by eating candies and ice-creams as snacks. Also, make sure you do not eat dried fruits, as they are high in bad sugars too.

Your snacks should include fruits and vegetables. Although fruits contain sugars too, these sugars are good sugars which have the added benefit of fiber and water.

Lunch and Dinner

In order to reduce sugar in your diet, you can safely consume meat, pizzas, pastas and vegetables in your lunch and dinner. You should, however, make sure that you cook these foods in your home, as ready-made foods contain relatively high sugar content. Also, make sure you do not use sauces which are high in sugars.

Drinks

Have you invited your friends for a party? If yes, then do not be tempted to offer soft drinks. Also, avoid wines and beers, as they too are high in sugars.

While drinking tea and coffee, you should not add normal sugar. Replace sugar with dextrose to enjoy tea and coffee without worrying about weight gain.

Some of the drinks which you should consume are unflavoured water, and unflavoured milk. They will give you less calories to burn and will fill you up with essential nutrients.

To conclude, avoid all the foods mentioned above, to prevent you from weight gain and other health issues. We know it can be difficult, but with patience and practice, you will learn to ignore your sweet tooth.

Chapter 11 – Read the Label

Brian was concerned that his weight was not going down despite his regular workouts. He was avoiding all that he was not supposed to eat. Despite being protective, however, his cholesterol level rose, and he gained a few extra pounds.

There was one major mistake, which Brian was making. He was not checking the nutrition label on the back of the products. Fancy packaging and a 'fat-free' label were used to attract him to buy the products.

It is this mistake which led to him gaining a few more pounds, instead of shedding them. It was this lack of knowledge which increased his cholesterol level. Therefore, for an effective weight loss, it is essential that you read the nutrition label before you buy any food product.

We know how confusing reading the nutrition label can be. With so many unknown terminologies, and confusing mathematical numbers, you may not want to glance at the back of the packaging.

Reading the food label, however, will help you make informed and healthy decisions. You will know how much nutrition the product will supply, helping you to make your decision. You will be able to limit your intake of bad fats and sugars if you read how much fats and sugars the food contains.

By reading the labels, you may be able to maintain your weight. You will know if the food you are buying contains high calories or not. Also, it will help you compare two products. When two foods look similar to you, make your decision by checking the quantity of nutrients each will provide.

Reading the nutrition label is essential as it can help you maintain your weight. It can also keep health issues like cholesterol at bay. You should not repeat Brian's mistake, and should start reading the labels, if you haven't already.

We know it may take a lot of your time to stop at each shelf, pick up a few products, and try to decipher the nutrition present. But, by practicing the tips in this chapter, you can master the art of reading labels.

Food labels are like table of contents. They tell you the amount of each nutrient present. They can also tell you what the food product is made of.

Here is an example of what a food label might look like.

Nutrition Facts

Serving Size 1 cup

Amount per serving

Calories 247   Calories from Fat 88

	% Daily Value
Total Fat 10g	15%
Saturated fat 3g	13%
Trans-fat	
Cholesterol 10mg	3%
Sodium 190mg	8%
Total Carbohydrate 39g	13%
Dietary Fiber 1g	5%
Sugars 22g	
Proteins 3g	

Vitamin A	5%	Vitamin C	2%
Calcium	4%	Iron	10%

Let us now analyze each component in detail.

Serving Size

Nutrition Facts
Serving Size 1 cup
Amount per serving

Calories 247   Calories from Fat 88

Serving Size

Serving size is the first thing you should look for. Serving sizes are standardized, making it easier for you to compare two foods. Serving size will tell you the amount which people usually eat.

Looking at the serving size is important, as it tells you the calories you are going to consume. The nutrient facts written will be true for the mentioned serving size. But, the entire packet might contain even more than the serving size mentioned. For example, the serving size at the label might be '1 cup'. The information written below on the label will tell you how much nutrients you will get for 1 cup only. The calorie level, in our label is 247.

But, for example, you bring the package home and find out that the whole packet contains 2 cups of food. Thus, if you eat the whole packet, you will double the nutrient intake, and will consume 494 calories. Therefore, make sure you check the serving size and the actual amount of food in the packet before you consume the whole of it.

Calories

Nutrition Facts
Serving Size 1 cup
Amount per serving

Calories 247   Calories from Fat 88

Calories

Checking the number of calories is another important thing to look for. It is especially important if you are serious about reducing your weight. Look at your labels and see how many calories they provide.

Looking at the calorie levels can help you decide between two products. Go for the products which will give you lower calories per serving, along with all the essential nutrients.

You should also look for calories from fat. Choose those foods which will give you lower calories from fats, as saturated fats and trans-fats can be harmful for your weight.

You should also note that if a package contains 40 or less calories per serving, then it is a low calorie food. A food will give you moderate calories, if it gives you 100 calories per serving. Also, 400 or more calories per serving is usually considered to be a high amount.

% Daily Value

Nutrition Facts

Serving Size 1 cup

Amount per serving

Calories 247   Calories from Fat 88

	% Daily Value
Total Fat 10g	15%
Saturated fat 3g	13%

% Daily Value

% Daily Value tells you what percentage of the daily recommended level of calories is included in the package. While calculating the percentages, it is assumed that an average person needs 2000 calories daily.

In our example, the calories you are getting from fat are 15% of the daily recommended level. This means that you will get 15% of your daily calorie intake from the fat the food contains. You should note that if the serving size increases, this value will increase as well.

Daily value will also tell you if the food is high or low in a nutrient. As a general rule, a daily value of 5% or less is considered to be low. Whereas, a daily value of 20% or higher is considered to be high.

Percentage daily value will also help you to make comparisons. When serving sizes are equal, you can easily see which product will give you a higher percentage or a lower percentage of a particular nutrient.

Fats

Total Fat 10g	15%
Saturated fat 3g	13%
Trans-fat	
Cholesterol 10mg	3%
Sodium 190mg	8%

Always check the percentage of fats (saturated and trans-fat), cholesterol and sodium before you buy a product. For a healthy weight loss, you should buy products which give you a low percentage of these 4 nutrients.

Saturated fats and trans-fats are bad for your weight. They can increase a few extra pounds in your bodies, and can increase the risk of having high cholesterol and high blood pressure. You should, therefore, limit these nutrients. Choose a product with low amounts of saturated and trans-fats.

Having a high percentage of cholesterol can also be bad for your weight and heart. Therefore, you should limit the level of cholesterol as well.

Sodium can be dangerous for your weight, as it can retain water in your bodies. This can give you a blown up look, and you will gain a few extra pounds. Thus, choose products with low percentages of sodium.

Carbohydrates

Total Carbohydrate 39g	13%
Dietary Fiber 1g	5%
Sugars 22g	

These are the nutrients which you should consume more. Carbohydrates can easily be found in the fruits, vegetables and grains. Dietary fiber, can be very important for weight loss, and should be consumed in a high amount.

Sugars can be of two types: natural and added. Look for the ingredients and see if the sugars mentioned here are added or natural. Added sugars are bad for you while natural sugars can be beneficial.

Thus, if the ingredients say 'fructose', then added sugars are included. You should then select a product with low value of sugars.

Proteins

Proteins 3g			
Vitamin A	5%	Vitamin C	2%
Calcium	4%	Iron	10%

Proteins

Proteins are beneficial for your weight loss regime. They should be consumed in a higher amount. However, make sure that the product offering proteins is low in saturated fats. There is no point in obtaining proteins from a product which will fill you up with bad fats, and will increase your weight.

Essential Nutrients

These nutrients too should be consumed in a greater amount. This is because they will help you maintain a healthy weight. They will also prevent you from various diseases. Therefore, look for products with high amounts of these nutrients.

You now know how to make an educated decision regarding the product to buy. But, there is more to the story. You may find some terminologies on the labels, which are necessary for you to understand.

Calorie free

If you find a product saying 'Calorie Free', don't be tempted to take the product without looking at all the other nutrients it is providing. A calorie free product does not contain zero calories. **Rather, they contain less than 5 calories.**

Fat-free and sugar-free

97

YOUR 'Lose Weight FAST the Natural & Healthy-Way DIET'

A fat-free or sugar-free label indicates that a very small amount of fat or sugar is included in the product. Generally, a fat-free or sugar-free product will contain less than 0.5 grams of fat and sugar respectively.

Fats

There are several other terminologies used regarding the amount of fats in the products.

- ▶ **Lean:** A product called lean contains less than 10 grams of fats. This includes 4.5 grams of saturated fats and 95 milligrams of cholesterol.
- ▶ **Extra Lean:** An extra lean product will contain less than 5 grams of fats, including less than 2 grams of saturated fats and 95 milligrams of cholesterol.
- ▶ **Low fat:** One serving of a low fat product will provide less than 3 grams of fats.

Cholesterol free

A cholesterol free product will provide less than 2 milligrams of cholesterol per serving

Sodium free

A sodium free product will give you less than 5 milligrams of sodium per serving.

Check the ingredients

In order to make healthy decisions regarding which foods to buy, it is important that you go through the ingredients as well. **Ingredients are listed in such a way that the ones added in large quantities are listed first.** Checking ingredients is important for weight loss, as you need to check whether bad sugars and bad fats are included in the product or not.

To conclude, we have told you the importance of reading labels. We have also given you tips to make healthy choices by looking at the labels. By practicing the above mentioned techniques, you can keep your weight at an even keel.

You can also lower your risk from diseases. The next time you pick something up from a shelf; make sure you read its nutrition label before adding it to your cart.

Chapter 12 – Count the Calories

Increasing proteins, reducing bad fats, and consuming carbohydrates are not the only things you should focus on to reduce weight. Perhaps the most important thing for you should be to count the number of calories you consume and burn off.

Calories are important for your body. They provide your organs with the energy to perform different functions. If you eat a few calories, your calories will be used up by your body. However, if you consume more than you need, then the calories can cause you to gain a few extra pounds.

Counting the calories is important. It will help you realize if you have eaten more calories than needed. Counting the calories, and managing the input and output amounts, can significantly help you lose weight.

Reducing your weight is all about checking the input and output of calories. If the calories you put in are greater than the calories you burn off, then you can gain weight. Similarly, if the number of calories you consume will be less than the number of calories you burn, then you will lose weight. Lastly, if your input and output levels are balanced, you will be able to maintain your weight.

This is the reason why counting calories is important. It will help you analyze your input and output calorie levels. You will then be able to reduce your weight.

For example, suppose you take in 3,000 calories throughout the day. But, because you were busy, you ended up burning 2,500 calories only. In this case, your input levels are greater than your output levels.

The extra 500 calories which you could not burn will remain in your body. They will then be stored as extra fat. This can cause you to gain extra weight.

3,000 – 2,500 = + 500

You will gain weight

On the other hand, if you consume 3,000 calories and burn 3,500 of them, you will lose weight. This is because your body will burn the extra 500 calories stored in your body.

3,000 – 3,500 = - 500

You will lose weight

Therefore, by counting the number of calories you input and burn out, you will be able to determine whether you can lose weight or not.

COUNTING INPUT CALORIES

We know how tiring this task can be. You may have to use your calculator several times. Or, you may have to use your brain for mental arithmetic. But, with some simple techniques you will be able to master this task.

Reading the nutrition label

Reading the nutrition label at the back of food packages should be the first thing you do to count your calorie intake. Nutrition labels will give you a fairly good idea about the calories contained in the food.

Through these labels, you can also look at the number of calories you will get through saturated and trans-fat. Reading labels can be of great help, because they will tell you exactly how many calories you have taken in through the food.

Before you count the calories, look at the serving size. The calories mentioned will be according to the serving size written on the label. For example, if the serving size is 1 cup, then the calories mentioned will be the calories you will gain if you consume one cup of the food.

However, the entire packet might contain 3 cups of food. So, if you consume the whole packet, you will get 3 times the calories mentioned. Make sure you count your calories by looking at the serving size on the label.

Food diaries

You can also keep track of what you have eaten by writing everything down in a diary. Don't just write what you have eaten; write the number of calories you have gained from each food too.

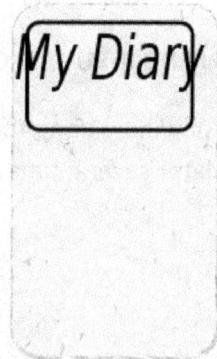

My Diary

This will be helpful, as at the end of the day you will be able to count the number of calories you have eaten in the day. Also, a diary will help you in cutting down a few foods if they have given you higher calories.

We know it can be a tiring job. You may not want to fill in your diary after a tiring day with kids or at the office. But, in order to lose your weight, this is an essential step.

Learn calories provided by common foods

If you yawn at the thought of taking out a calculator every time you eat something, then try learning some standard numbers. You can learn calories given by common foods in order to avoid calculations.

For example, if you drink orange juice and eat eggs in your breakfast every day, you can learn the calories they provide. In this way, you will not have to calculate the calories eaten the first thing in the morning.

In the same way, if you like to eat a particular salad every few days, learn the calories provided by the salad. This will give you enough time to concentrate on other important issues. You will then not have to worry about calculating calories while you are working.

Online calorie counter

In order to save yourself from the hassle of counting calories yourself, you can use an online calorie counter. There are various websites on the internet which can calculate your daily calorie intake for you. But, for this, you will have to maintain a food diary. You should know what foods you have eaten throughout the day before the website can count the calories for you.

These calculators are particularly important when you are dining out. When you eat out at a restaurant, you do not know the amount of calories your meal has provided. It may be weird to ask the chef to tell you the calories included in the food. In that case, it will be wise to count calories through these online calculators.

CALCULATING THE CALORIES YOU BURN

Counting the number of calories taken in is not the only thing which is needed. In order to lose weight, you also have to count the number of calories you burn.

There is one little problem here. You can easily take in a lot of calories through different foods, but you will not be able to burn them off easily. As an example, if you eat one M&M candy, then you will have to run an entire football field to burn the calories gained from a single candy. This means that if you eat a few more candies, you will have to run a few miles to burn the calories gained from just a few candies.

Burning off calories is therefore a tough task. This is the reason why we are asking you to count the calories taken in and burnt off.

Counting the number of calories you can burn seems like a daunting task at first. This is because you burn calories even when doing small daily chores. You may also not know how many calories you will burn when you exercise.

But, we are here to make your lives easier. Below is a list of a variety of exercises. We will tell you how many calories you will burn in each of the exercises mentioned below.

Before that, you should know how many calories you will need to lose 1 pound of weight. Generally, **you will have to burn 3500 calories to reduce your weight by one pound.** It may seem impossible to achieve at first. But, with practice, you can easily achieve your target.

Swimming	Swimming at a moderate pace for around 1 hour can help you burn 560 calories.
Running	If you run for 1 hour, then you will burn 700 calories.
Walking	Walking at a moderate pace for 1 hour will help you burn 350 calories.
Biking	Biking will help you burn 280 calories in an hour if you do this exercise at a speed of 10 miles per hour.
Stair climbing	Stair climbing will burn 450 calories in an hour.
Weight lifting	If you do weight lifting for an hour, then you will burn 250 calories.

Basic metabolic rate

You burn calories not just by exercises, but through simple movements as well. You even burn calories when your heart beats and when your lungs expand during breathing. Around 70 percent of your total calorie burning comes from daily bodily movements.

But, how to calculate the number of calories burnt by bodily movements? **Calculate your basic metabolic rate** to know the number of calories you burn when you sit back and do nothing.

You will find a number of websites to calculate your basic metabolic rate. This rate will also help you determine the calories used during simple household chores or office work.

Generally, the **calories you will burn through simple movements will be 20 percent of your basic metabolic rate**. By remembering this rule, you will be able to calculate the calories taken out through household and office chores.

Calculate the calories you burn through simple movements and bodily functions using your basic metabolic rate. You can then count the number of calories you burn through exercises with the help of the above information.

After you count the total number of calories you have managed to burn at the end of the day, subtract it from the calories you had put in to see whether you have gained weight or lost a few pounds. Through this you will be able to realize whether your exercise regime is sufficient or not. It will also enable you to see whether there is a need to cut down input calories. It is only by managing your input and output levels that you will be able to gain a smart physique.

Chapter 13 – Supercharge Your Metabolism with 10 Fat Burning Foods & Drinks

Your body is a great machine. Whether you are eating, breathing, drinking, or sleeping, your body needs to constantly burn calories to keep you going.

Whether you eat your favourite fruit, or you dine out, your body will break down the food into energy. This is the energy that fuels our organs.

The process of breaking down the food to provide energy is called metabolism.

There are several factors that affect the metabolism of any given person, such as height, weight and body composition (the amount of muscle you have), the frequency of the meals you consume, personal diet, activity levels, genetics, and stress levels. While the rate of metabolism slows down for many reasons, the 3 most common causes are:

1.   loss of muscle because of not enough physical activity

2.   the tendency of the body to cannibalize its own tissue because there is not enough food energy to sustain it

3.   the decrease of physical activity that comes naturally with old age.

Keeping your metabolism supercharged is the answer to keeping the extra pounds from making it to your stomach, hips and thighs. If your metabolism is in high gear, it can burn the extra calories instead of storing them as fat.

So how do you speed metabolism up? How do you supercharge your metabolism to help you burn more calories and fat? Here are a number of unique and interesting strategies to do just that!

Cayenne Pepper

Cayenne Pepper is usually used as a medicine and in cooking. But, do you know that it is a great tool to boost your metabolism?

Cayenne Pepper has the power to increase your metabolism up to 20 percent. It will also help you in burning the excess fat stored in your body. The spice in this pepper comes from a compound called Capsaicin.

Capsaicin is the true agent which helps you increase your metabolism. Have you ever felt your body getting warm after you eat some spices? This is what Cayenne Pepper does. It will increase your body's temperature, which your body will then try to cool down.

Now, while cooling down the heat produced by the pepper, your body will burn calories. There is also good news for anyone who has excess fat in the body. Eating Cayenne Pepper will affect proteins, which in turn will break down your excess fat.

Forget about the runny nose and the teary eyes. Include this pepper in your daily diet for a faster metabolism, and a slim look. You can easily add Cayenne Pepper to a lot of your dishes.

However, if you do not like spicy food, try Cayenne Pepper powder. It will make your dishes less spicy and will boost your metabolism. You can also take a capsule of Cayenne Pepper powder daily to get the same benefits.

Try including Cayenne Pepper in your daily diet, and feel your metabolism increasing.

Salsa

Another great tool to speed up your metabolism is salsa. Salsa will boost your metabolism by 15-20 percent, and can give you a slim body shape. Salsa too contains Capsaicin.

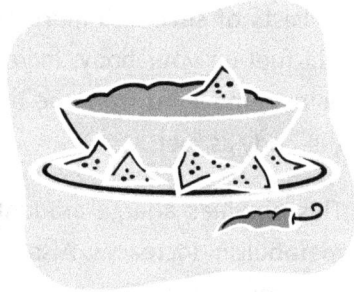

When you eat a hot salsa, your body gets heated up. You will burn calories when your body tries to decrease the gain in temperature. Your excess fat can then reduce, and you can lose weight.

The hotter your salsa is, the better it is for you. This is because a hotter salsa will burn more calories. Also, while improving the metabolism, salsa can help you feel satiated. If you eat salsa in your meals, you may end up eating less food.

Apart from an increase in metabolism, salsa will help in the digestion process. If you regularly eat salsa, your digestive system can improve, and hence you will be able to lose weight in a healthy way.

Add salsa in your daily meals and boost up your metabolism. The good news is that you can eat salsa with almost everything. You can easily eat salsa with eggs anytime. Have it with chicken, meat and vegetables and enjoy a slim figure.

Green Tea

Green tea too can boost your metabolism. It also has the ability to reduce your fat and weight. Whether hot or cold, the particles in those tea bags are full of benefits.

Green tea is able to increase your metabolism because it consists of several important antioxidants. These antioxidants will fuel up your body, increasing your metabolism. Green tea helps remove fat from the body, so that the fat can be used by the body as fuel.

This provides a large amount of energy for the body, and our metabolism increases. Also, your body can lose extra fat during the process as well.

Benefits of green tea have been proven by research. Also, it is widely known that drinking green tea daily will help boost your metabolism by 4 percent daily.

Green tea is a great tool for weight loss as well. Drinking tea on a regular basis can help remove the excess fat stored in your bodies. Generally, you should drink three to five cups of green tea daily if you want to reduce extra pounds.

We know drinking three to five cups can be too much for you to drink in a single day. But, try different favours of green tea for a variety. You can also tune into your favourite food channel and learn how to make a green tea soda.

Apple cider vinegar

Apple cider vinegar is an amazing metabolism booster. By increasing your metabolism, it can help you lose weight.

It increases your metabolism by increasing the amount of iron absorbed in the body. When absorption of iron gets high in your bodies, your body utilizes oxygen in an efficient way. This leads to an increase in the metabolism.

Apple cider vinegar can also reduce your appetite. It is best to take apple cider vinegar before meals for an effective weight loss. Drink apple cider vinegar 3 times a day before meals. You should take around 2 teaspoons of it with 1 glass of water. This can significantly help you with weight loss. Also, it can boost your metabolism.

Potent cocktail

It is not just the foods which can help you increase your metabolism. Some cocktails can boost your metabolism as well. One such booster is tomato juice.

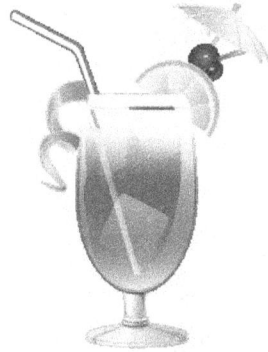

Try a glass of tomato juice with some hot sauce and horse radish. You can also add some fresh lime to make the drink more appealing. Drinking this juice in the morning will help you start your day with an energy boost.

Celery

Celery is an amazing metabolism booster. It is also called a negative calorie food. This means that the numbers of calories spent while eating celery will be greater than the number of calories gained.

This is the reason why celery should be a part of your daily diet. It will boost your metabolism, and give you a slim shape. Eating celery can also fill you up with fiber and vitamins too.

Fibers and vitamins can help reduce your hunger. This can result in your weight being reduced. Include celery in your salads and foods and see your metabolism boosting.

Brussels sprouts

Here is another way to increase your metabolism: start eating Brussels sprouts. Brussels sprouts are famous for a number of health benefits. They can also reduce your weight if you eat them regularly.

Brussels sprouts are low in cholesterol and high in fiber. These fibers will help you fight several diseases, such as cancer. Fibers can also make you feel full and satiated, helping you to reduce your weight.

Weight loss benefits of Brussels sprouts have also been proven by research. Therefore, it is important that you include them in your diet. You should, however, look for green Brussels sprouts. This is because the greener they are, the better they will be.

Brussels sprouts are also full of proteins. If you want some change in your protein diets, try eating Brussels sprouts in your meals, to get loaded with proteins.

Spinach

Do you remember Popeye the sailor? Recall that he used to eat spinach to get an instant energy boost. Spinach is actually a source of great strength. This is the reason why Popeye used to beat the big Brutus with ease after eating spinach.

The reason why spinach can fill you up with energy is that it is full of iron. Iron increases the working power of your haemoglobin, resulting in an instant energy gain.

Spinach is also low in calories. It will give you energy, without increasing your weight. Spinach contains vitamins too. These vitamins will make you healthy during your weight loss regime.

Spinach is also loaded with calcium. Calcium is famous for making your bones stronger. If you want to reduce your weight, while keeping yourself healthy and energetic, go for spinach every day.

Grapefruit

Grapefruit is an essential metabolism booster. It contains several vitamins, especially vitamin C, and can fill you up with energy and health.

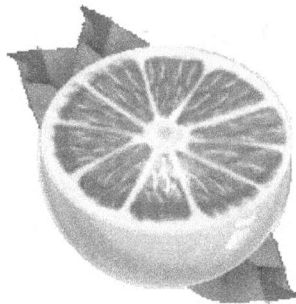

Grapefruit is also a good tool to reduce your weight. It helps in the digestion process by breaking down the proteins easily. Also, it can help the body burn fat at a faster rate.

Therefore, drink a glass of grapefruit juice daily to get an energy boost. Drinking the juice in the morning can speed up the weight loss process. Drinking it in the morning can also empower your liver and stomach, so that they can burn off the fat easily. Try drinking its juice with some cinnamon to get a different taste.

Fatty fish or flax oil

Do not get scared by reading the word 'fatty fish' and 'oil'. Fatty fish will not make you fat. Neither will the oil. In fact, they both can help you reduce your weight.

Fatty fish and flax oil contain omega-3 fats. These fats are the 'good fats' which are vital for your body. Thus, consuming them may not only reduce your weight, it will also give you lower calories and higher energy.

To conclude, all of the foods mentioned above are essential to boost your metabolism. In order to get a slim physique, it is important that you consume these foods. Be creative, and try making different dishes out of them.

Section 2

Weight Loss Benefits for You and Your Family

Do you remember the story we told you about Edward in the first introduction? Edward had gained weight because he was ignorant about his health and weight. He was being classified as obese by the doctors, but he paid little attention to it. He continued with his sedentary lifestyle, and his unhealthy eating habits. This resulted in a lot of problems for Edward.

It all began when he was in a middle of an important discussion with a client regarding a new merger. While talking, he suddenly felt his heart feeling heavy. With the passage of time, the pain in the left part of his chest grew. The pain extended to the back and spine as well.

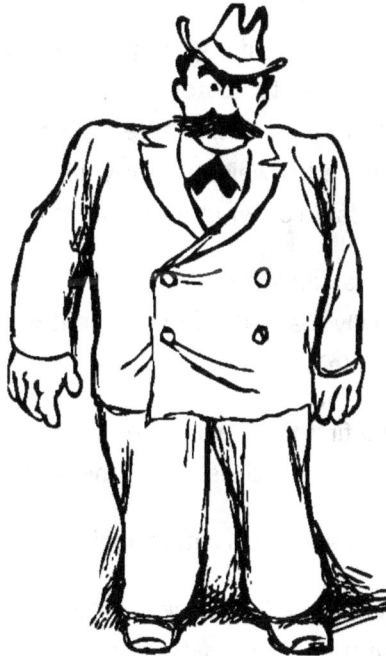

He started feeling exhausted. He could not breath properly, and it felt as if the pain was about to kill him. Seeing the blood draining away from Edward's face, his client reacted immediately.

Edward was rushed to the hospital where the doctors treated him with utmost care. It was then revealed that Edward had faced his first heart attack.

He was hospitalized for a few days. But, after he came back home, his health never recovered. His blood pressure was usually high and his heart often felt heavy. Initially, he used to come back early from his job. But as the health deteriorated, he started missing his work. Gradually his health worsened to a point where he could no longer continue with his business.

The business which was started with so much passion was now fading away. Seeing his life going downhill, he started getting depressed. With time, the depression continued and every aspect of Edward's life was severely affected.

Seeing his life getting worse, Edward's wife left no stone unturned to restore Edward's health. Edward was taken to various doctors, where all he heard was that he needed to reduce his weight. Nearly all the doctors told him to cut down the fat in order to free himself from his various diseases.

It was after these visits that a realization dawned on him. He finally realized that his weight was the culprit of all the mess in his life.

The first thing which he did was to join a gym. He started doing regular exercises, so that he could burn off the extra fat stored.

He changed his eating habits.

He started practicing portion control, and reduced his consumption of saturated and trans fats.

He decreased his intake of sugary foods, and increased his consumption of fruits, vegetables, proteins and all the essential nutrients.

In short, Edward followed all that is written in the first section of this book.

While his weight was reducing, his blood pressure was also reducing. He no longer had a heavy feeling in his heart, and his depression was under control as well.

Weight loss had a lot of benefits for Edward.

While he strictly followed a weight loss regime, he regained the lost pleasures in his life.

He re-established his business, and his financial condition improved.

He reconnected with his family and everyone started to enjoy their family time together.

In short, Edward's life changed after he started reducing the extra pounds stored in his body.

You can gain exactly the same benefits if you are overweight and you follow a healthy weight-loss regime. While weight gain can be a curse, weight loss can be a blessing.

With a bulging belly you may never feel good about yourself. However, when you see yourself losing your excess weight, imagine the pleasure that you will gain.

It is not just a healthy body which you can achieve if you follow a weight loss regime. In fact, there are various other health benefits of weight loss which you may not know. While the last section gave you comprehensive tips to reduce your weight, this next section will cover all the additional benefits which you can achieve if you sincerely follow all the weight-loss tips.

This section may leave you surprised about the hidden benefits of weight loss. You may be surprised to know that if you reduce your excess weight, you can decrease the risk of heart diseases, as well as help prevent diseases as dangerous as cancers and infertility.

If you follow all the weight loss tips, your life can be much healthier. You should reduce your consumption of unnecessary calories. This is because these extra calories can convert into fat, creating pressure on your organs. This pressure can sometimes be so huge that your nerves may burst and you may get have a stroke.

You should also reduce your consumption of bad sugars, in order to help protect yourself from various diseases such as diabetes. It is when you limit the intake of all the unhealthy foods that you can see your weight being reduced.

Now, once your weight starts reducing, you may notice a lot of positive changes in your life. You may be more energetic and less lethargic. Your metabolism will boost up, helping you to effectively concentrate on all aspects of your life.

Also, experience the blessing of weight loss and see your life improving. Like Edward, if you have a problem of being depressed about your weight or financial condition, you can see your depression fading away as you enjoy your new slim look.

If you were to choose between a healthy lifestyle and a life full of diseases, what would you choose? We are sure you would prefer to stay healthy, active and fit. Read the next section to see how weight loss can result in additional benefits for you and your family.

Every third adult in the USA suffers from the problem of high blood pressure. **It is one of the most common problems in the world right now.** High blood pressure can damage your heart, kidneys and other vital organs of your body.

Normal blood pressure is above 80 and below 120. You should frequently check your blood pressure to see if it is normal. This is because it usually damages the organs of your body without showing any symptoms.

Causes of high blood pressure

Perhaps the main reason for high blood pressure is **weight gain**. If you are overweight, you may have experienced high blood pressure. Your heart may have felt heavy, and at times you may have had to stop your work because of the terrible condition you were in.

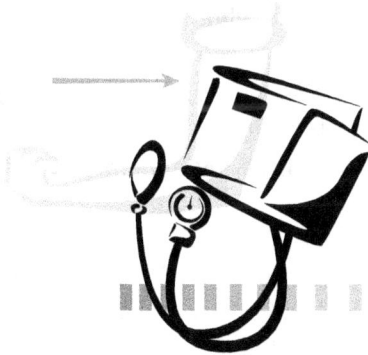

This is a grave consequence of over eating. Gaining weight will increase the chances of high blood pressure.

A study was conducted for 44 years to study the relationship between obesity and high blood pressure. It was found that out of all the men who experienced high blood pressure, 26 percent of them were overweight.

Also, out of all the women who had problems of high blood pressure, 28 percent of them were obese.

After reading this, we are sure nobody would deny the fact that with obesity high blood pressure may occur. This is because when you are overweight, you may consume more junk food and saturated fats. These fats are harmful for your health, as they store as excess fat in the body.

The excess fat stored can then put pressure not just on your heart, but on your kidneys and arteries as well. This can create problems for your heart to function properly. Your blood circulation can be negatively affected, and your blood pressure can rise.

Moreover, if you consume a lot of calories, while you do not burn enough of them, the difference of calories will stay in your body. These extra calories will be converted into fats again, and can harm the body in the same way.

Therefore, to live a healthy and happy life, it is extremely important that you cut down your calorie and junk food intake. Exercise is essential here too, because it can burn off the extra fat stored.

Kidney disease is also one of the main causes of high blood pressure. Kidneys control the amount of blood and fluid in our bodies. When kidneys do not work perfectly, the amount of blood increases in our bodies and so does the force required to push the blood through the whole body.

Polycystic Kidney Disease

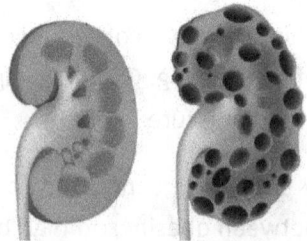

Kidneys often malfunction when you are overweight. This is because being overweight can build up excess fat in your bodies. This excess fat can stick to several organs, including your kidneys, creating a hindrance in the pumping of blood.

When your kidneys are under stress, your heart can also be under stress. Therefore, you should stop eating all the junk foods you like. This is because they can build up fats to pressurize your kidneys, and your blood pressure can shoot up.

Hormonal imbalances can also lead to an increase in your blood pressure. Release of certain hormones can increase blood pressure. This is because they disrupt the flow of blood.

Weight gain is often the cause of these hormonal imbalances. Here we have given you another reason to reduce your weight.

High blood pressure is extremely dangerous for your health, as it can sometimes lead to death. High blood pressure can also put stress on your arteries, and thus they can get damaged.

Perhaps the most affected part of your body will be the heart. Since your heart is the machine which pumps the blood, a higher blood pressure can lead to malfunctioning of your heart. The increasing pressure inside the heart may cause the size of the left part of your heart to increase. In severe cases, extra strain can lead to heart failure.

High blood pressure will not just affect you physically; it can put you in a **mental torture**. Imagine you are in the middle of cooking dinner for your family or guests, and you suddenly feel terrible. Your heartbeat shoots up and you can no longer stand in the kitchen. Your heart and your body feel heavy suddenly.

What will you do with your family and guests then? You will certainly not be able to attend to them.

This can lead to a mess in your family life. Your husband and your kids may leave without breakfast, as there may be no one around in the morning to make breakfast for them. Seeing you in a hospital can also make your family feel depressed, and they may not be able to live a normal life.

Now what if you are a working woman, or a working man? Now imagine yourself in the middle of an important meeting. Imagine yourself on the verge of making a very good deal. What if your blood pressure shoots up suddenly? Will you be able to convince the other company to invest in your project in the same way? Most probably, your deteriorating health may not allow you to continue with the same tactics.

This is what high blood pressure can do to you. It can affect your whole life, and can even lead to death. Therefore, for a healthy and happy life, it is extremely important that you control high blood pressure.

Since weight gain is the main cause for high blood pressure, **reducing your weight** can help protect you from this fatal disease. When you lose a few extra pounds, your chances of getting higher blood pressure can significantly reduce. Out of all the benefits you will get from reducing your weight, lower blood pressure is perhaps the most important one.

You may no longer have extra fat stored in your body. Your arteries may no longer have any extra pressure. Your heart may not malfunction, and therefore, your overall life can significantly improve.

Let us now tell you some of the **foods**, which will not only help reduce your weight, but can help to control your blood pressure.

- Vegetables
- Fruits
- Nuts and beans
- Low fat dairy products
- Poultry, fish and lean meat

You should include these foods in your daily diet. Eating these foods can reduce your weight, and can also provide you with an additional benefit of lower blood pressure.

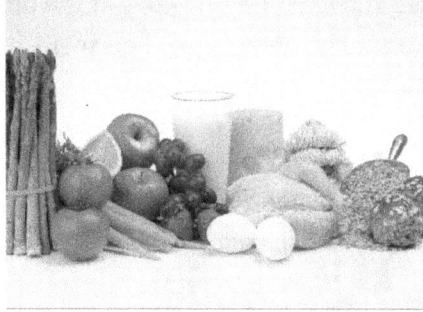

You should also practice portion control techniques here, and should eat according to the recommended serving size. Also, drink lots of water to have a happy heart.

Another thing which you need to monitor in your diet is salt or sodium. High sodium can also lead to high blood pressure. Therefore, it is important that you do not consume salty foods. Here are some of the ways to reduce sodium in your diets:

- Increase spices in your foods and cut the amount of salt used.
- Make sure to rinse canned foods. They often contain sodium in them.
- Use fresh meat and poultry, instead of frozen. This is because frozen foods are often high in salt contents.
- You can use cinnamon, chilli powder, sage and parsley instead of salts in your foods.

These are some of the ways to ensure that your sodium level stays at an even keel. When you reduce your sodium consumption, your body may not gain weight. Hence, you could be saved from high blood pressure.

Another way to avoid high blood pressure is to engage in sports. We know after a tiring day at the office or at work, you may not want to go out and jog. But, there are some activities which you can easily do.

- Take a brisk walk.
- Sweep your driveway, or shovel the snow.
- Wash your car.
- Walk to the store instead of driving.
- Take the stairs.
- Ride a bike.
- Park at the end of the parking lot and walk.
- Go for a swim.

The list is endless. The trick is to just get started and do SOMETHING!

These can all help you lose weight, and can lower your blood pressure as well.

Weight gain is the main cause of high blood pressure. High blood pressure can be dangerous for your health and devastating for your personal and professional life. We have also told you how reducing your weight can give you a more peaceful life. This is because reducing your weight can help you get a lower blood pressure. This in turn can make your life happier.

Therefore, the next time you shudder at the thought of going through a tedious weight-loss regime, read this chapter again. Read all the problems which you are likely to get from being overweight. Then imagine how easy and happy your life will become if you lose a few extra pounds.

Chapter 15 – Protect Your Heart from Diseases

Your heart is one of the most important organs of your body. It is a small machine which supplies blood to each and every cell of our body.

It is important that you take care of this helpful machine and prevent it from diseases. This is because a sick heart can truly jeopardize your life.

One of the reasons why your heart may feel sick is your increasing weight. Extra fat stored in your body may hinder your heart's functioning. However, if you lose weight, that can help to prevent the harmful effects of an ill heart.

The most common disease that overweight people get is Coronary Heart Disease (CHD). CHD is caused when an increase in your weight leads to an increase in the production of a waxy substance. This waxy substance sticks to your heart and blocks it from pumping blood.

This waxy substance also enters your arteries which supply blood to the heart. This substance sticks to the walls of the arteries and disrupts the flow of blood.

These are the arteries which are responsible for supplying blood to your heart. When these arteries get clogged, your heart does not get enough supply of oxygen rich blood.

When the supply of blood to your heart gets disrupted, you might get high blood pressure and in severe cases, a heart attack and a heart failure.

CHD is also caused by high levels of cholesterol. Do you know where cholesterol comes from? It comes from the saturated

126

fats you eat. When you consume saturated fats, your liver converts the saturated fats into cholesterol.

The cholesterol is carried in the blood where it plays an essential role. Although cholesterol is needed by the body, a high level of bad cholesterol can be dangerous. A high level of bad cholesterol in your blood can result in the clogging of arteries.

Cholesterol can stick to the walls of the arteries and can disrupt the flow of blood. When the flow of blood is disrupted, you may be at an increased risk to get CHD. So, do you see the link between CHD and weight gain?

You eat saturated fats, you gain weight, your cholesterol level increases, the bad cholesterol sticks to the walls of the arteries, arteries get clogged, blood flow is disrupted, and you get CHD. Here is an illustration to help you understand better.

saturated fats

↓

Weight gain

↓

cholesterol increases ▶ stick to the walls

blood flow disrupted ▶ strain on heart

▲ ↓

arteries clogged

▲ ↓

Heart Diseases

CHD

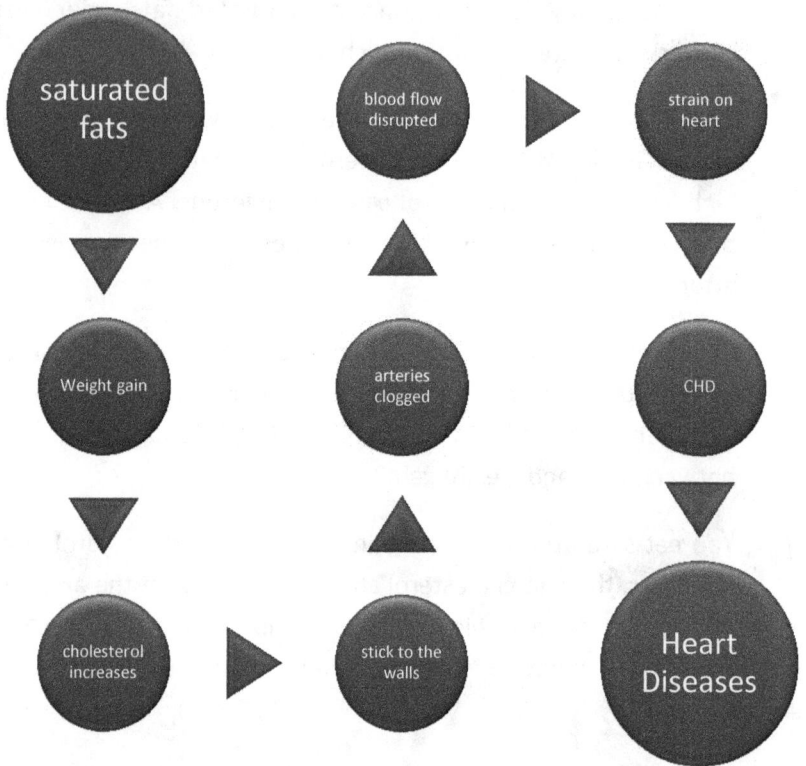

Now, do you see the harmful effects of weight gain here?

You may have felt your heart feeling heavy sometimes. This can be a consequence of your high weight. When you gain a few extra pounds, you are at an increased risk for Coronary Heart Disease (CHD).

When your heart's ability to pump blood decreases, you can get a heart attack. In severe cases, you can get a heart failure as well. Therefore, it is important that you lose excess weight to help prevent a heart failure.

Heart failure is something to get scared of. This is because it is a long term disease and can worsen with time. Heart failures occur when the ability of the heart to pump blood efficiently decreases. In severe cases, a heart failure can be fatal.

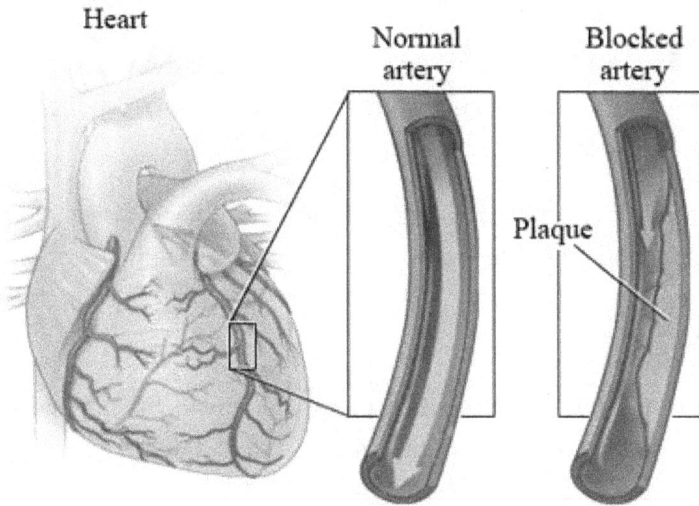

A heart failure can occur because of many reasons. But, the most common reason is weight gain. Weight gain and heart failures are directly proportional. As your weight increases, extra fat gets stored in your bodies. This fat produces cholesterol, which can then get inside the blood and clog the arteries.

Clogged arteries are not able to carry blood around easily. This can then significantly reduce your heart's ability to pump the blood around the body. You can experience high blood pressure and a heart failure.

Another consequence of heart failure and CHD is a heart attack. A heart attack also disrupts your overall wellbeing. It can also prove to be fatal, thus it is essential that you lose your excess weight so that the risk of a heart attack decreases.

Have you been able to identify the real culprit behind all these heart diseases? Yes, it is your weight. Your weight can be the agent who can trigger these heart diseases in the body.

It is extremely important that you reduce your excess weight, so that you can help protect yourself from the paralyzing effects of these diseases on your life.

Here we have a list of the negative effects of heart diseases, and weight gain. By reducing your weight, you can reduce potential heart diseases, as well as protect yourself from the side effects too.

Protect yourself from dizziness: Gain in weight is positively correlated with heart diseases. And, heart diseases are positively correlated with dizziness. When your heart stops functioning in the best possible way, your overall health can be affected. Blood supply to the other parts of the body, including the brain, can reduce significantly. This can hinder their functioning.

As a result, you can suffer from light headedness and dizziness. You may not be able to actively perform your job. Be it the household chores, or your job, your performance can suffer.

Therefore, to protect against this from happening, take time out to burn the fats, and reduce your intake of calories. By reducing your weight, you can live a happy life, and can prevent yourself from the constant feelings of dizziness.

Protect yourself from heart attacks: A heart attack can lead you to be hospitalized for several days. This can hamper your personal and professional life. Even if you stay at home and suffer from a minor heart attack, you may not be able to do simple household chores.

You may not be able to cook for your family. Your kids may suffer badly as no one may be there to make breakfast for them in the morning. Your house may be in a mess, because you may not be in a position to clean your home.

If you are a working woman or a working man, you may not be able to go to your office. Even if you suffer from a minor heart attack, your doctor will probably advise you to rest for a few days. This might lower your performance at your job.

Another benefit of reducing your weight is that when you help to protect yourself from heart diseases, you will be at a lower risk for heart attacks.

Protection from constant coughing and wheezing: Constant coughing and wheezing is a consequence of heart diseases, and hence, weight gain. A heart failure can sometimes result in some water being added in your lungs. This added water can be the cause of constant coughing and wheezing.

Imagine yourself sitting in the middle of the meeting of the board of directors. If you are overweight and you suffer from heart failures, chances are that you will get a constant cough attack as well. Imagine how embarrassing it will be if you couldn't stop coughing while an important point is being discussed.

For some time the other directors around may ignore the disruption created by the coughs. But, when these coughs will not stop after a few minutes, everyone may start getting irritated from your presence. In severe cases, they might even ask you to leave.

Therefore, to prevent yourself from these embarrassing moments, start working on your weight today. When your weight is reduced, you can decrease the risk of heart failure, and hence, no embarrassing coughs too. Your life can be peaceful and everybody will love your presence.

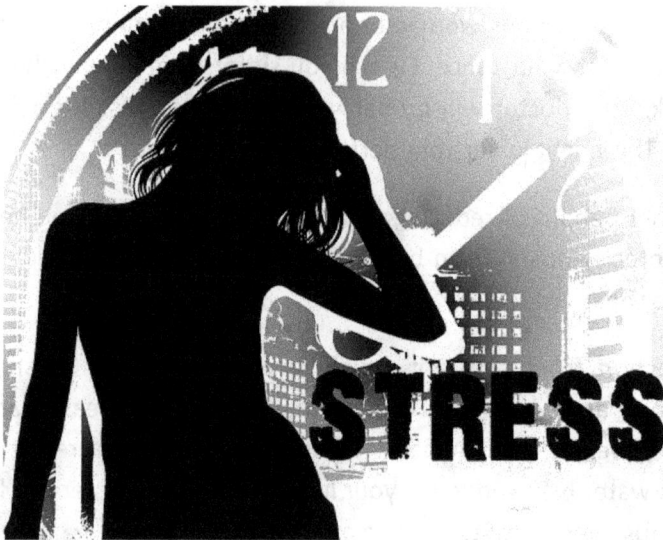

Protect yourself from stress: Another consequence of weight gain, and thus, heart diseases, is that you are more likely to develop depression. It is proven through research that people who suffer from heart diseases can also suffer from stress and depression.

Stress and depression can have a lot of side effects on your personal and professional lives. They can spoil your family relationships, especially your relationship with your spouse and children.

Heart diseases can be extremely dangerous for your life. It is important that you reduce your excess weight while also decreasing your chances of getting heart diseases. It is through a reduction of weight that you can help to prevent yourself from stress and depression also.

Other benefits of reducing weight and heart diseases are:

- ▶ Prevention from chest pain, which is a consequence of heart diseases.
- ▶ Prevention of fatigue. Fatigue is caused by malfunctioning of the heart too.
- ▶ Prevent yourself from the problem of shortness of breath. This is a problem which most people suffering from heart diseases have to go through.
- ▶ Prevent yourself from an early death. When you are overweight, the chances are higher that you will get heart diseases. This can increase your chances of heart attacks, strokes, and heart failures, which can be fatal sometimes.

We are sure everybody wants to live a life free from these diseases. We are sure nobody wants to die an early death. Therefore, it is **important that you protect yourself from heart diseases. Here, weight loss is the most important prevention.**

Fortunately, weight loss is a great help to reducing the risk of heart diseases.

Take time out from your schedule, and set up a regular exercise program. Also, the next time you go shopping, make sure you do not buy anything which is likely to increase fats in your body. Start working on your weight to get the benefits of a happy and carefree life.

Chapter 16 – Stroke Prevention

Stroke is the third leading death cause around the world. Worldwide, 15 million people suffer a stroke each year. Out of these, 5 million die whereas 5 million people are disabled for life. However, you can help prevent strokes by reducing your weight.

Stroke is caused by a blockage of blood supply to the brain or is a cause of bleeding in brain tissues. Effects of strokes vary according to the injured part of the brain. Weakness, difficulty in speaking and seeing, and loss of senses are some of the effects of strokes.

Types of strokes

Normally, there are two types of strokes: Ischaemic strokes and Haemorrhagic stokes. Ischaemic stroke is the most common type of stroke. It accounts for about 80 percent of all strokes around the world. One of the main causes of Ischaemic stroke is high cholesterol levels and diabetes.

When arteries around the head or neck become too narrow to carry blood cells because of cholesterol decomposition, they form blood clots. These clots can block the blood flowing to the brain which can cause stroke. In some cases, clots dislodge

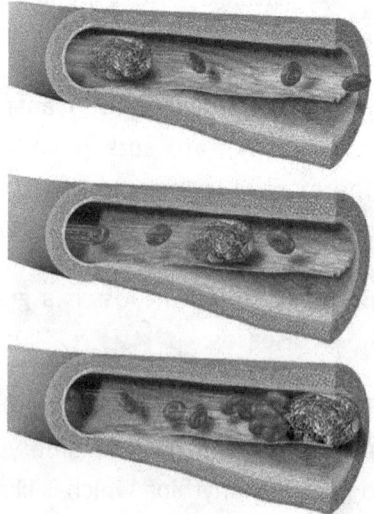

and are trapped in arteries near the brain. This is the major cause of Ischaemic stroke.

Haemorrhagic strokes are caused when a blood vessel in the brain bursts and leaks the blood inside the brain. This can damage the brain cells around the blood. Unexpected increase in blood pressure may also cause death or unconsciousness.

Risk of strokes

Certain factors increase the risk of strokes in people. Age is one of the most important factors. People of 65 years or above are more likely to have a stroke. However, about a quarter of strokes affect younger people.

Moreover, if you have a family member who suffered from stroke, your chances of having a stroke are higher. And people who previously suffered from stroke also have higher chances of having a stroke.

Causes of strokes

Being overweight is one of the major causes of strokes. As it increases your blood pressure and cholesterol level, and can cause diabetes, all these are main causes behind strokes.

Being obese increases your blood pressure which is the major cause of a stroke. About 12.7 million out of 15 million strokes worldwide are caused due to high blood pressure. This is because high blood pressure damages the blood vessels of your body and damages arteries of your brain.

When you are overweight, or obese, you are likely to take in a lot more calories. Also, you may not be following a proper exercise regime. If this is the case, the extra calories which were not utilized in your body will be stored as extra fat.

The fat can gather around your organs, creating a hindrance in their functioning. The blood may not reach there properly, and your blood pressure may rise. In some cases, the pressure can be so high that the arteries are damaged.

Because of damaged arteries, clogs can be generated in your body that block the blood supply to your brain. It also causes Haemorrhagic stroke as damaged arteries of the brain can burst and leak blood in your brain.

Obesity can also result in high cholesterol levels, which then can cause you to suffer from strokes. Cholesterol is a fat produced by the liver, and is vital for normal body functioning. However, increased cholesterol levels increase the chances of strokes as excess cholesterol is deposited in the arteries of your body.

This blocks the flow of blood to your brain or creates a blood clot which may cause Ischaemic stroke. Foods with high saturated fats, eggs, meat, pies and hard cheese are some of the foods that contain high levels of cholesterol.

When you are overweight, or obese, you are likely to consume the foods which are high in saturated fats. This then becomes a reason for strokes.

If you are overweight or obese, you are at an increased risk for diabetes. Diabetes is a condition in which the pancreas does not produce enough insulin to control the blood sugar level. In some cases, the body may stop responding to the insulin released by the pancreas.

Weight gain is one of the main causes of type-2 diabetes, one in which the body does not respond to insulin production. If you develop diabetes because of being overweight, then your blood sugar level may shoot up.

This shooting up of the blood sugar level contributes to a stroke. So, did you see the connection between weight gain and strokes here? You gain weight, you can get diabetes, your blood sugar level can shoot up, and you can suffer from a stroke. If you manage your weight, you may be able to help prevent stokes from occurring.

You may also suffer from the problem of sleep apnea if you are overweight. Sleep apnea is a sleeping disorder in which you momentarily stop breathing while sleeping. You may also start snoring. Having sleep apnea can put you under a lot of risk of suffering from high blood pressure and strokes.

You may also suffer from the problem of enlargement of the left side of the heart if you are overweight. It is a serious condition which is caused by high blood pressure and weight gain. When the left side of the heart is enlarged, there are higher chances that you might get a stroke.

There are also chances that your increased weight may cause a metabolic syndrome in your bodies. This metabolic syndrome can be dangerous for your health. In severe cases, metabolic syndrome leads to heart diseases and strokes.

So did you see how your extra weight can lead you to strokes through different channels?

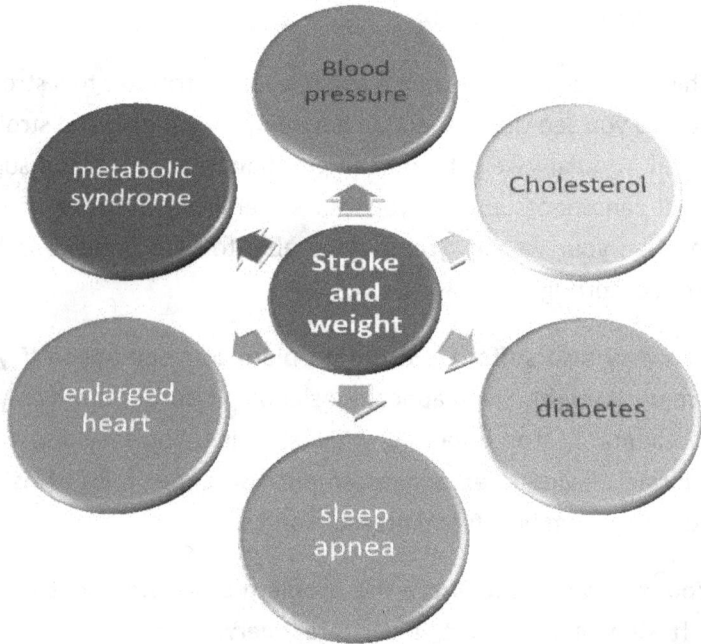

Hence you should control your weight, so that you can reduce your risk of getting a stroke. This is because strokes can be perilous. It can greatly affect all aspects of your lives.

When you get a stroke, the brain damage may not allow your body to function properly. Some of the body parts might get paralyzed.

You may not be able to carry out your everyday jobs if a part of your body is paralyzed. You may have to leave your job, and your career may come to a halt.

If you are a working woman, then imagine the distress it may cause you if you cannot take care of your house. Being paralyzed can also make you dependent on someone. In short, strokes can jeopardize your whole life.

It is extremely important that you prevent yourself from stroke. You can help prevent strokes just by managing your weight. It has been proven by research, that **reducing a few pounds can decrease the risk of stroke by more than 50%.**

How to reduce the risk of strokes through weight management?

Exercise

You can control your weight by doing regular exercise. Regular exercise can burn off the extra calories. When there are no extra calories, your heart can stay in better health, reducing the risk for strokes.

It has been proven by research that exercising 5 times a week can significantly reduce the risk of strokes.

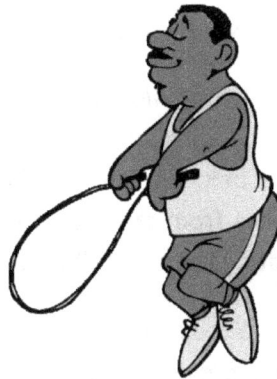

You can go out for a walk early in the morning with your friend, or you can exercise at home. You can also join a gym to burn off the extra calories. Try swimming and cycling for a change. They will not only help manage your weight, but can keep your heart happy.

Avoid eating saturated fats

A healthy diet, coupled with an exercise regime is the key to lose weight. You should eat a diet which is low in calories. To make your diet a healthy one, avoid eating foods containing saturated fats.

Eating less saturated fat means you have less fat stored in the body. When you will have less fat stored, your heart will have less problem in carrying out its functions. There will be less chances of getting strokes.

While avoiding saturated fats, try adding omega-3 fatty acids and unsaturated fats in your diet. These are the foods which will help you lose your weight, and can help protect you from strokes.

Add vegetables and fruits

Fruits and vegetables are an excellent way to keep strokes at bay. Eating fruits and vegetables in your daily weight-loss diet will help you burn off the extra fat. It will also help protect your heart from other type of diseases. Keep your heart healthy by eating healthy fruits and vegetables.

Here are some of the foods that you should add in your diet to help prevent strokes:

- ▶ Beans
- ▶ Antioxidants, such as onions and carrots
- ▶ Potassium-rich fruits, such as bananas
- ▶ Oats and almonds
- ▶ Low-fat milk
- ▶ Foods rich in magnesium, such as barley
- ▶ Salmon

These foods are known to provide you with all the essential nutrients that your body needs. While doing so, they will ensure that the total calorie intake is minimized. These foods will help you lose fat. Once the fat is reduced, your chances of stroke will decrease as well. Also, the essential nutrients in these foods can help ensure that your heart stays healthy and happy.

Weight loss is truly a blessing, as losing your weight can enable you to keep the most important part of the body healthy.

Do you love chocolate cakes and ice-creams? Most people do! Do you know that eating lots of them can lead you to weight gain and diabetes? Perhaps not.

Reducing your weight will not only give you the benefit of looking slim, it can also help prevent you from getting diabetes.

Diabetes is a disease which affects your blood sugar level. It can be caused when your body stops producing enough insulin, or when your body stops responding to the insulin. Diabetes in fact, is a metabolism disorder.

What is insulin? Insulin is a hormone which is released by the pancreas. The pancreas is a small gland which is very close to the stomach. The insulin released by the pancreas helps control the sugar in our blood.

You get glucose from food and your liver. Glucose provides energy for muscles and tissues, and is important to consume. Whenever we eat anything, our pancreas automatically discharges insulin to control the level of glucose entering the blood.

You get diabetes when your pancreas cannot release enough insulin to control the amount of glucose in the blood. Or, your body may be producing insulin, but your cells will not respond to it. Since there is no hormone present to control the amount of glucose in the blood, your blood sugar levels will shoot up.

When you practice a weight-loss diet, you will consume fewer sugars. This will allow you to help control your diabetes in a better way. So, here is **another benefit of weight loss: you can help manage your diabetes.**

Diabetes is a very prevalent disease. A large part of every country's population has diabetes. Diabetes can be dangerous sometimes. This is because when glucose builds up in the blood your body loses glucose through urine. You will keep on losing the main source of fuel, while your cells will not get glucose for their functions.

When your blood contains high levels of sugars, your nerves get damaged. Also, there are chances that high sugar levels may lead to stroke and kidney diseases. It is important that you manage your diabetes, so that you live a healthy lifestyle.

Types of diabetes

There are three main kinds of diabetes

- ▶ Type-1
- ▶ Type-2
- ▶ Gestational

Type-1 diabetes is caused when the pancreas cannot produce enough insulin to maintain the sugar levels. Some of the cells inside the pancreas are destroyed, which restricts it from releasing enough insulin. Therefore, people who suffer from type-1 diabetes have to inject insulin in their bodies to live properly.

Type-1 diabetes can occur at any stage. Whether you are young or old, you can develop type-1 diabetes.

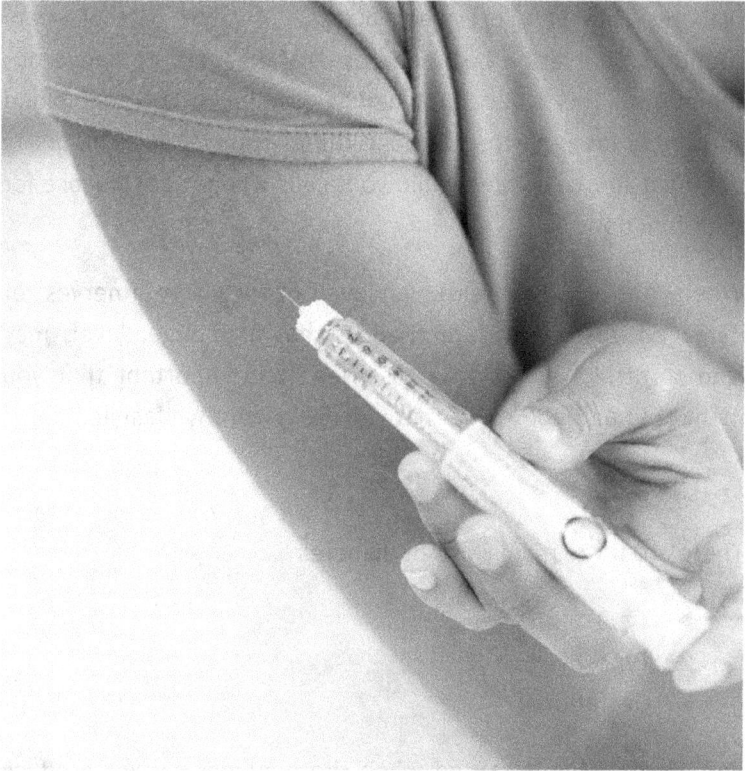

Type-1 diabetes is mostly inherited through genes. If your parents or your close relatives have type-1 diabetes, you are at an increased risk of developing diabetes too. But, you need not get upset here. This is because if you practice a weight-loss diet, your risk of getting type-1 diabetes will significantly reduce.

Consuming high amounts of sugars is one of the reasons for weight gain. This high consumption of sugar can increase your risk of getting type-1 diabetes. However, if you reduce the quantity of sugars consumed, your weight can significantly reduce, and your diabetic risk can be minimized.

If you have some chocolates and sugary foods in your refrigerator, give them away to a kid, as they can aggravate your situation. This is especially true when you carry the genes for type-1 diabetes.

By controlling your weight you may be able to prevent your family from a burden of buying insulin daily. Daily insulin buying can sometimes be expensive for families. Thus, it is important that you **save calories**, so that you can **save some pennies** too.

If you already have type-1 diabetes, being overweight can aggravate the situation. The extra fat stored in your body will make it difficult for you to control your type-1 diabetes. It is important that you start cutting down your weight, so that you can manage your type-1 diabetes in a better way.

Obesity and type-2 diabetes

Type-2 diabetes is the most common type of diabetes. In this case, the pancreas still produces insulin, but the ability of the body to respond to insulin decreases. This is known as **insulin resistance.** When this happens, the sugar level in the blood rises, leading to the pancreas producing even more insulin.

No matter how much insulin is produced, the body does not respond to it. Tired and worn out, the pancreas can stop producing insulin after some years. This can lead to an increase in the blood sugar levels and the person can get type-2 diabetes.

There are several reasons for insulin resistance including,

- ▶ Being overweight, and
- ▶ A bad diet

Obesity is the major cause for insulin resistance. Your body releases certain chemicals when you are overweight. These chemicals distort the body's ability to respond to insulin released by the pancreas. Being overweight can also distort your metabolism, and you are more likely to develop this metabolic disease.

Being inactive will also increase your chances of getting type-2 disease. Also, if you follow a bad diet, you are more likely to develop this disease.

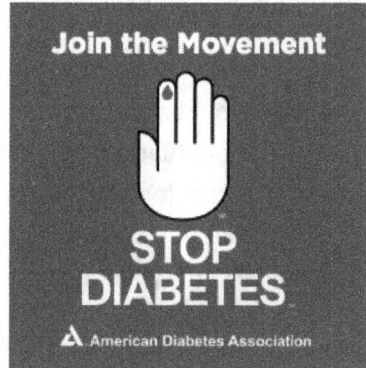

Join the Movement

STOP DIABETES

American Diabetes Association

What do we mean by a bad diet? This is a diet consisting of 'bad sugars' and 'bad fats'.

Consuming a large amount of sugary foods, coupled with zero activity during the day, can significantly raise your blood sugar levels. For example, your chances of getting type-2 diabetes increase by 22% when you consume your favourite sodas.

If you do not control your weight and diet, you can develop insulin resistance. This insulin resistance must be prevented; you may otherwise have to stay dependent on insulin injections for the rest of your life.

It is therefore important that you reduce your weight, so that you reduce your chances of getting diabetes. If not prevented, insulin resistance can lead you to several other bodily impairments. There are chances of developing Metabolic syndrome and infertility if you do not control your weight, and hence insulin resistance.

You might be thinking that you will have to work hard to reduce your weight to prevent diabetes. However, studies have shown that a small quantity of weight loss will have a multiplier effect, and your risk for diabetes will decrease even more.

> **If you reduce 10% of your weight:**
>
> ► Your glucose levels will decrease by 30-50%
> ► Risk of developing diabetes will decrease by 50%

Did you read the last point in the box above? It says your risk for developing diabetes will be halved if you reduce your weight by just 10%. This means, if you decrease your weight by 20-30% you will decrease the risk of developing diabetes even more. Having strong genetic inheritance is an exception though.

Start working on your weight now. Cut down your consumption of fats and sugars, as these are the culprits of diabetes. Here are some tips for you to follow.

Do not starve to lose weight:

Reading the above box can make a few people excited to lose weight. They will then ask friends and family members for some tips to reduce weight. Since friends and family members are not usually nutritionists and doctors, chances are that they will misguide you.

They may tell you to completely eliminate certain foods from your diet. In some cases, they might even tell you to starve so that you can lose weight.

This is a dangerous thing to do, however. You need small quantities of all kinds of foods, including sugars. By depriving your body from these foods you can worsen the situation. It can create problems for your body to manage your blood sugar levels.

In case you are taking insulin injections, starving may cause the insulin to not work properly. It is not advisable that you starve to lose weight. Follow a proper diet plan, one that allows you to eat all kinds of food, but in a limited quantity.

Proper diet plans may take time to reduce weight. But, they will be healthy in the long run. They will help prevent and manage your diabetes.

Do not skip insulin injections

If you are already diabetic, do not skip your insulin injections while following a weight-loss diet. This is because skipping insulin can worsen the problem. When you skip insulin, your sugar levels may get so high that you may suffer from a coma.

Since inactivity can also lead to weight gain and diabetes both, **plan out an exercise regime today**. Set a target weight, and do the appropriate amount of exercise to reduce your weight.

So, you see, weight loss is like a blessing. Firstly, it can give you a slim figure like those celebrities. Also, it can help protect you from different diseases, one of them being diabetes.

What is the first thing that comes to your mind when you hear the word cancer? It is perhaps a fatal disease. Cancer is one of those diseases which cause significant harm to our bodies.

Cancer is caused when there is an abnormal growth of our cells. These damaged cells replicate themselves and spread quickly to different parts of the body. These cells accumulate at one place, causing tumors to develop.

Cancer can be dangerous, as these rapidly growing cells interrupt our bodily functions. They spread from one organ to the other and damage the healthy tissues there. They create problems for our organs, which then cannot perform their tasks properly. Our organs get destroyed, which may even lead to death.

There are many types of cancers. Be it stomach cancer, blood cancer or skin cancer, all types of cancers are scary. They all damage our bodies. Some of these cancers can be treated if diagnosed at an early stage. However, the later the diagnosis, the harder it gets to cure the cancer.

Causes of cancer

Cancers are caused when the cells rapidly replicate themselves. This replication can be caused by various reasons.

DNA Damage

Damage of the DNA can cause cancer. This damage can then cause our cells to replicate uncontrollably. This damage can sometimes be controlled by our body. However, in case when the damage is not corrected, our body can develop cancers.

149

Heredity

Cancers can be inherited from families. If your family has a history of developing cancers, you may be at an increased risk for developing cancers too. You may inherit a faulty gene from your parents, which can then cause the cancer cells to replicate themselves rapidly.

Viruses

You can develop cancer if you catch certain types of viruses. This does not mean that you will catch cancers like you catch flu from other people.

Certain viruses can interrupt the working of your cells, causing them to get damaged. These damaged cells then multiply themselves and can cause cancer. For example, you may develop liver cancer from hepatitis B and C viruses.

Weak immune system

If you possess a weak immune system, then you are at an increased risk for developing cancer. This is because a weak immune system cannot fight with the viruses and infections that attack us on a daily basis. These infections and viruses can lead to damage of the cells, which then turns into tumors and cancers.

Obesity and risk of cancer

There is a strong correlation between weight gain and cancer. You are at an increased risk for developing cancers if you are overweight.

Around 20 types of cancers are caused because of being overweight.

When you are overweight, your body releases certain hormones. These hormones may interrupt the working of your cells and may damage them. This damage can then lead to many types of cancer.

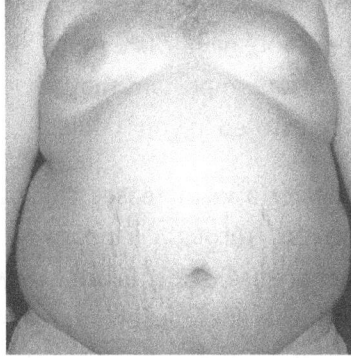

If you are overweight from a very young age, then the risk of getting cancers are higher. It is not just the childhood weight which is problematic; weight gain during adulthood also increases the risk for developing cancer. Also, rapidly changing weight may also trigger cancer in your body.

Here are some of the types of cancers that may develop if you are overweight:

- ► Kidney cancer
- ► Pancreatic cancer
- ► Gallbladder cancer
- ► Liver cancer
- ► Thyroid cancer

These are just some of the cancers which can be developed from being overweight. **Obesity can also lead to bowel cancer.** In fact, it is the main cause of bowel cancer. When you consume a lot of calories, and do not burn enough of them, the extra calories can get stored around the stomach as fats. This extra fat can then create problems for your stomach to work properly. They may cause damage to the tissues and cells, leading you to bowel cancer.

This has also been proven by research. If you are overweight, then you have 50% more risk of getting bowel cancer. It is therefore important that you cut down your calories so that fat is not stored in your bodies.

Obesity also increases the risk of breast cancer. It has been proven through research that if you have undergone menopause, and you are overweight, then the likelihood of you getting breast cancer is very high.

If you gain 4–22 lbs (2-10 kg), and have passed menopause, then there are 30% more chances of you getting breast cancer. Also, your chances of getting cancer will increase by 45% if you gain 55 lbs (25 kg) of weight. It is important that you manage your weight, and reduce it, to help protect yourself from this dangerous cancer.

We are telling you this so that you can manage and control your weight. Cancers are perilous diseases. Once you develop a cancer, it takes a lot of effort to control the growing cells. You may have to undergo expensive treatments to cure cancer.

You may have to have chemotherapies and radiotherapies. In chemotherapy, cancerous cells are destroyed using drugs. These drugs are effective in destroying the cancerous cells. However, while doing so, they destroy the healthy cells and tissues as well. Your immune system will drastically reduce, and you can become unhealthy.

Radiotherapy is another treatment which you can take. In radiotherapy, radiations are used to kill the cancerous cells. But, here again these radiations can destroy the healthy cells as well. In both of the treatments, your health can be affected. Also, you may start getting bald, as your hair may start falling off.

We are sure you do not want to see yourself in this situation. **Prevention from cancer** is the best way to avoid getting into these situations. In order to help protect yourself and your families from the burden of cancer, **start reducing your weight**.

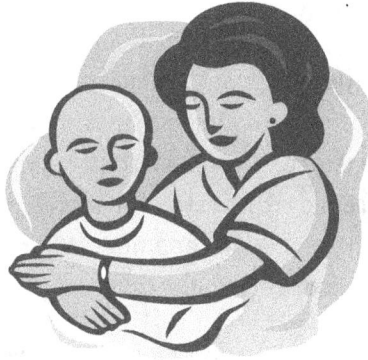

Since weight gain can cause cancer, **weight loss can prevent it**. Weight loss comes with lots of benefits for your health, and cancer prevention is just one of them. Studies have shown that weight management significantly reduces your risk of developing cancer.

If you lose 20 pounds, your chances of getting cancer will decrease by 11%.

This ought to have made you excited about losing weight. Start working on your weight from today, and help keep cancers at bay.

By reducing your weight, you may make your life significantly better. This is because people who have cancers usually live miserable lives. They can no longer look after their families and kids, and have to leave their jobs. In case where a person is the breadwinner, leaving the job deteriorates the financial condition of the family. Also, medications and treatments may decrease the savings to zero.

However, when you reduce your calorie intake you can significantly reduce your risk of getting cancer. You can live a happy and healthy lifestyle if you cut down a few pounds. You can be able to be at your best in your home, your job, and your school.

Therefore, stop making plans with your friends to go out and have junk food at restaurants. Start making plans for exercise instead. A good exercise regime, along with low-calorie food can reduce the extra fat stored in your body, especially the fat around your abdomen. **When this fat decreases, so does your risk of getting cancers.**

Also, when you reduce your weight, **you may not have to face insulin resistance.** Insulin resistance is a condition in which the body stops responding to the insulin produced. Insulin resistance is caused by weight gain, and can lead you to some types of cancers.

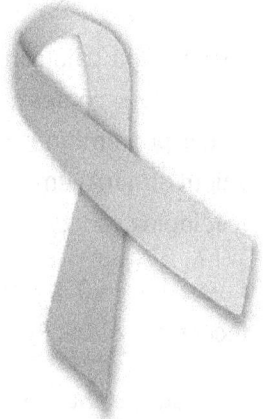

Doing exercise to reduce your weight can also strengthen your immune system. When **your immune system is stronger**, your body will be in a better position to fight off the replication of cells. Your risk of cancer can thus reduce.

Some of the cancers, such as breast cancer, are caused by disturbance of some hormones. These hormonal disturbances can be caused by weight gain. Consequently, if you reduce your weight, there may be **no hormonal disturbance**, and you can help better protect yourself from the risk of getting cancer.

Reducing weight to help prevent cancer may be a tough job, but one that is certainly worth the effort. You have to reduce the consumption of certain foods and increase your daily exercise levels.

Here are some research statistics related to exercise and cancer prevention:

- The risk of getting breast cancer can reduce by 30-40% if you follow a moderate exercise regime and workout for a minimum three hours per week.
- The risk of getting colon cancer can reduce by 40-50%, if you exercise regularly.
- The risk of getting uterine cancer can reduce by 38-46% if you follow a moderate exercise regime.

Join a gym, and get ready to jog the first thing in the morning. You should also try to increase consumption of healthy foods, such as foods containing mega-3 fatty acids. Decrease your consumption of unhealthy and junk food. Change your lifestyle a bit, and get physically active. You can get a slim figure, and can also help protect you from the trauma of getting cancers.

Chapter 19 – Reduce Infertility

Are you one of those who are overweight and suffer from the problem of infertility? Potential good news! Infertility can be reduced by weight loss.

Infertility is a problem in which you cannot conceive. You are not alone if you suffer from this problem. Approximately 10% of couples in the United States suffer from this problem.

It is not just women who face the issues of infertility; men too can suffer from the problem. In some cases, the causes of infertility cannot be determined, but in most, the cause can be diagnosed.

Risk factors of infertility

Here are some of the things that can increase your risk of having infertility. These are the things which you should try to cut down on if you want to have kids.

▶ **Being overweight:**
   If you are overweight or obese, then there are high chances of you suffering from infertility. The extra weight creates hindrance for many parts of the body. It also creates problems for the female and male organs.

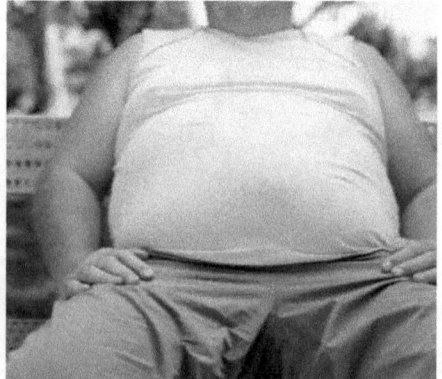

Thus, in order to reduce the risk of not having children, it is essential that you reduce your weight.

▶ **Being a vegetarian:**

If you are a vegetarian, then you may not be consuming enough iron, folic acid, zinc and vitamin B-12. Deficiency of these nutrients may create problems for the fertilization of eggs. Hence, consume these nutrients if you aren't already.

▶ **Not exercising:**

Living an inactive life can create many problems for a person. One of them is infertility. Whether it is men or women, they both are at increased risk of facing infertility if they live a sedentary lifestyle.

▶ **Over exercising:**

While not exercising is bad for health, over exercising can be dangerous too. If you are a woman and you exercise extensively, then there are chances that your reproductive system may get damaged. Hence, if you are exercising to lose your weight, make sure you do not over exercise.

Besides the reasons mentioned above, there are many other reasons such as stress and alcohol consumption, which may increase your risk of infertility.

Reducing infertility by reducing weight

Since being overweight increases your risk of not conceiving, reducing your weight decreases the risk. You should maintain a healthy weight, so that your wish of having children can be fulfilled.

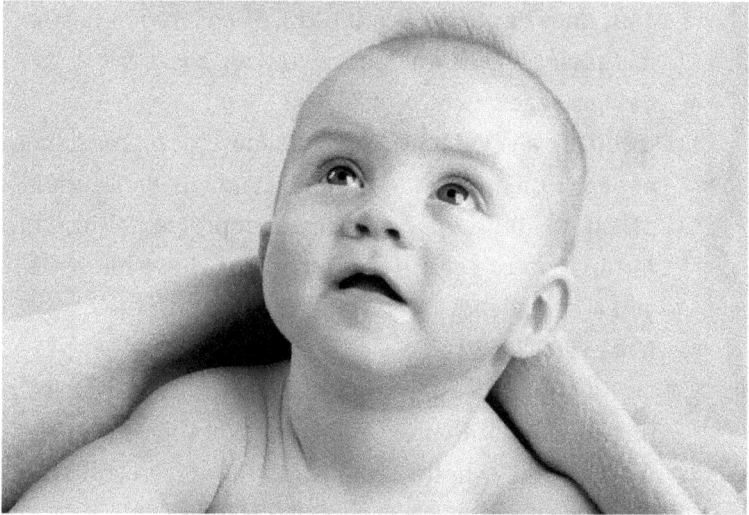

A body mass index (BMI) in the range 19 – 25 is an ideal BMI for women who wish to increase their fertility. If you have a BMI above 29, then you should reduce your weight to increase your fertility.

For men, a BMI of around 29 is ideal if they are facing fertility issues. If your BMI is above 29, then you should try and cut down a few extra pounds.

By reducing your weight you will hopefully be able to conceive. You can then feel the joy of having children. Also, you may not have to take expensive fertility treatments. The solution may be right there at your doorstep. Step out of the house and start exercising moderately to reduce weight, and hence infertility. Make sure you do not over exercise though.

Also, reduce your consumption of saturated fats, and increase your consumption of unsaturated fats. No matter how much the sugars appeal to you, reduce your consumption of sugar so that you can lose weight.

Eat a balanced diet, one which is full of nutrition. You should consume foods with zinc, iron and vitamin B12, especially if you are a vegetarian. Also, while eating out, make sure you reduce your consumption of oily foods.

If you reduce your weight, you may get the happiness of being parents. Your stress level may also significantly reduce. When a couple cannot conceive, they can undergo a lot of stress.

By reducing your weight, you may be able to save yourself from the stress of not having children. You will hopefully conceive and will be able to play with your kids.

Chapter 20 – Decrease Osteoarthritis

Examine the elder patients coming in for a treatment in a hospital, and you may be surprised to know that a lot of them are coming in to deal with the pain of osteoarthritis.

Osteoarthritis is one of the most common diseases in the elder generation. It is a disease of the joints in which the joints wear out.

You may also be surprised to know that this disease is the main reason for many people's disabilities. In this disease, the joints in your bones get damaged. This results in your bones getting injured. You may suffer from severe pain, and may not be able to move your bones at all.

Your bones and joints are likely to be damaged when the

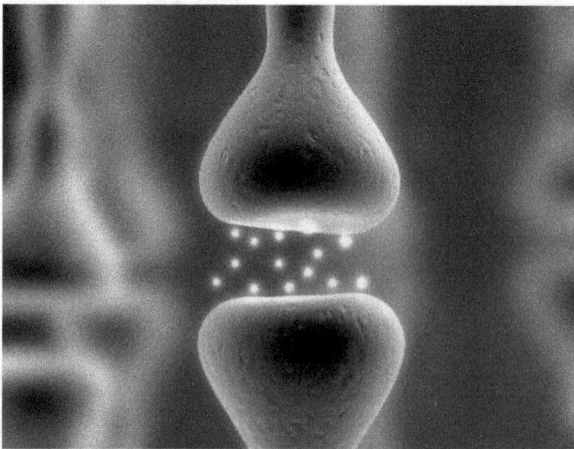

cartilage withers and becomes weak. Just like a lubricant in a machine, cartilage allows swift movement of your bones.

But what happens when the lubricant in the machine dries out? Machine wears out over time because of friction between the parts. You also hear squeaky noises while the machine runs.

This is exactly what happens with our bones in osteoarthritis. The cartilage, which was acting as a lubricant, deteriorates, and the bones become rough. They will rub against each other, and can destroy the tissues around the bone.

Hence, the rubbing and tearing will cause the bones to wear out over time. This can result in extreme pain. Also, with those cracking sounds coming out of your bones, you may sound like a machine whose parts have not been lubricated.

You will mostly find this disease in people who are more than 40 years old. You will learn in this chapter that weight loss can be an effective prevention for osteoarthritis.

Symptoms

Osteoarthritis usually affects the joints of knees, hands, spines and hips. If you develop osteoarthritis, then you may not feel extreme pain during the initial days. However, as you grow old and the disease develops, the symptoms can become extreme. Some of the symptoms that a person may experience are:

- ▶ You may hear a cracking noise while you move your hands, or knees.
- ▶ You may experience swelling around your joints.
- ▶ You may suffer from extreme joint pain.
- ▶ In severe cases, the joint may not be able to work at all. This can result in a disability.

These symptoms can be disturbing for a person. The pain and the suffering may not allow you to enjoy your twilight years.

Also, the disability can make you dependent on someone. It is essential that you help protect yourself from this disease.

Before we go on to tell you the ways to help protect yourself, let us tell you some of the major causes. These are the factors which can increase the risk of having the disease. Once you know them, it is important that you reduce these risk factors.

Risk factors

Weight gain

Weight gain can be dangerous. It brings along an obese physique, and some dangerous diseases. Osteoarthritis is one of them. **It is an established fact that a high body weight can lead to osteoarthritis.**

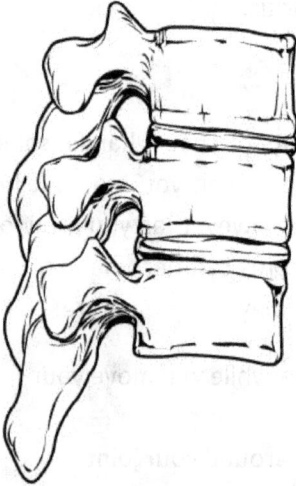

Normal vertebrae   Bone loss amplifies curvature

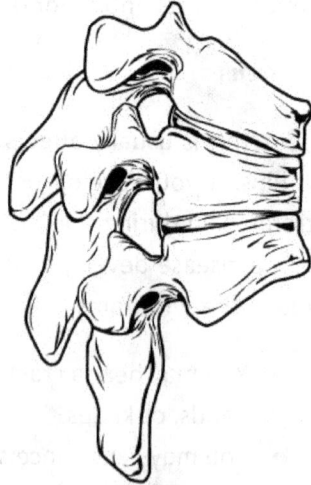

Why do you think weight gain can cause osteoarthritis? It is simple. When you gain a lot of calories, you can build up excess

162

fat in your bodies. You can gain weight, which puts extra pressure on every part of your body. This extra pressure is felt by the bones as well, which can lead to the damage of the cartilage.

Your weight can damage the bones of your hands, knees and hips especially, increasing your risk of osteoarthritis. Various researches have confirmed this point as well.

You can also gain weight when you take in more calories than you burn off. This may come from a lack of exercise. Less physical activity can also lead to osteoarthritis.

When you exercise, your bones move, and their working improves. However, when you do not exercise, the opposite can happen. How do you think a machine will work if it has not been used for a long time? It will not work efficiently, right? Same is the case with your bones. When you do not move them regularly, they may become rusted and damaged.

Lack of nutrition

Just like a machine needs oil to move, your bones need certain nutrition to make them strong. If you follow a diet which is low in essential nutrients, then you are at an increased risk for developing osteoarthritis.

By essential nutrients we mean fruits, vegetables, fish, and lean meats. Your bones also need certain vitamins and minerals, such as calcium, vitamin D, and vitamin C to make your bones strong. However, if your diet lacks these nutrients, then your bones may not become strong.

They can get weak over time, and their efficiency may reduce. As your age increases, you may experience pain in your bones. Here at this point, you are highly likely to develop osteoarthritis.

Heredity

Heredity is also a strong risk factor. If your parents or grandparents have suffered osteoarthritis, then it is more likely that you will get the disease too.

There are some genes which are responsible for manufacturing cartilage in your bones. However, if you inherit defective genes from your parents or other family members, then your cartilage may not be able to develop properly. It is when the cartilage is least developed that you can get the disease.

Joint injury

A joint injury can also lead you to osteoarthritis. An injury in your joints can weaken your bones, or can damage them permanently. In some cases, the alignment of the bones may be disturbed. This can become the reason for developing osteoarthritis.

Thus, if you have had a severe accident in the past which had damaged your bones, start feeding your bones with lots of nutrition so that you can help prevent the onset of osteoarthritis.

Age and gender

Age and gender are the strongest risk factors. As you grow older, your bones automatically weaken. On top of that, if you have a high body weight, and you have been feeding yourself with junk food, your chances of getting osteoarthritis will be very high.

Gender plays a role here too. Before the age of 45, men are most likely to develop osteoarthritis. While after 45, women are at an increased risk for developing the disease.

Therefore, if you want to reduce your chances of being disabled when you grow older, start reducing your weight, and improve your nutrition.

Prevention of osteoarthritis is essential. This is because it can jeopardize your life. With damaged bones and severe pain, your life can become challenging and hard.

In severe cases, your bones may damage to a point where you can be disabled. This is when life can become miserable. You may need an attendant or a nurse to help you with your tasks. You may not be able to go out, and you may not enjoy your favourite places.

In old age, most want to retire from work and enjoy their life. But, with severe pain and disability, this dream of having a comfortable old life may vanish.

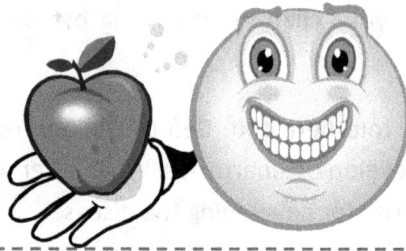

> **The good news is that even a little weight loss can be beneficial.**
>
> **Even if you lose just 10 pounds, you will greatly reduce the risk of osteoarthritis.**

It is necessary that you protect yourself from this disease so that you can enjoy your twilight years.

Weight loss will also decrease your chances of osteoarthritis even if you have inherited the defective gene. Thus, even if your parents have this disease, you need not worry. This is because by exercising and reducing your weight, you may be able to keep osteoarthritis at bay.

How can weight loss help you with osteoarthritis?

You can reduce weight by eating the right type of food, and by exercising to burn off the calories. These are the two essential tools which can also help you reduce weight and osteoarthritis.

Exercise

Exercise is perhaps the best thing which you can do to reduce your chances of getting osteoarthritis. Exercises can strengthen your muscles, and hence, the muscle around your bones can become stronger.

When the muscles around the bones are stronger, your bones will be better protected. Also, exercising can increase the flexibility of your joints. Protect your joints from getting rusted by moving your joints during the exercises.

You can easily go out for a walk to exercise. Wear some comfortable shoes, call your neighbours, and enjoy the beautiful sunshine by jogging and walking in the parks nearby.

You can also walk on the stairs more often to get your joints moving. Instead of taking the elevator, take the stairs so that you can increase the flexibility of your joints.

You can also exercise in the water. Go swimming, as swimming can be a lot of fun, and can greatly enhance the strength of your bones.

Nutrition

While reducing your weight, you should be eating foods which are healthy and low in calories. This is exactly what you need to reduce osteoarthritis. Eating lots of vegetables and fruits during your weight loss diet will provide strength to your weak bones and joints.

Also, eat foods which are rich in omega-3 fatty acids. Omega-3 fatty acids will not only help you reduce your weight, but can also power your bones and joints.

You should also ditch all the junk food which you may have been consuming regularly. This is because junk foods, and foods with saturated and trans-fats, will fill you up with excess calories. They can provide more weight while giving you less nutrients. A higher weight can then trigger the onset of osteoarthritis.

Thus, reduce your meals out and instead dine in with your family. Include vitamins and calcium in your daily diet, and work on a more healthy body and healthy bones.

So, did you see how easy it is to help protect yourself from a disease as dangerous as osteoarthritis? Reduce your excess weight by exercising, and by eating a healthy diet.

Chapter 21 – Get Rid of Back Pain

'Ouch, my back hurts!' You probably have heard this statement from your friends, especially if they are overweight. If you are overweight too, you might have experienced back pain as well. Back pain is a very common complaint.

More than 80% of adults face back pain at least once in their lives.

Back pain can often be the reason for your visit to the doctor. It can also be the reason for your absence from work. Hence, it is essential that you control and prevent it as much as possible.

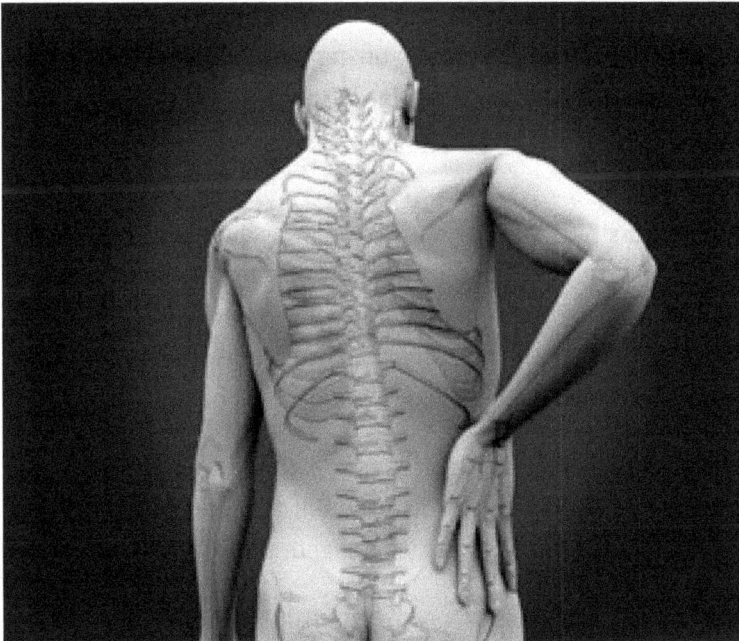

You will shortly see that if you lose excess body weight, that it can be very helpful for reducing and possibly controlling back pain.

While experiencing back pain, you may experience inflammation in your back as well. You may feel pain, starting from the upper part of your back, down to your legs. You may also experience numbness in the lower part of your body.

While back pain can often be temporary, if it persists then you should immediately contact your doctor.

Causes of back pain

Your back is made up of several bones, which help you move and bend with flexibility. However, if these bones experience stress and pressure, you can experience pain in your back.

While you may experience temporary back pain if you move and sit with poor body postures, you can get a serious back pain if these postures become a regular part of your life.

Stress and strain

Stress and strain on your back are one of the major reasons for back pain. You are most likely to strain the bones and muscles on your back, if you regularly lift heavy objects. Also, if you lift things up with poor movement and postures, then your bones may get strained, leading you to severe back pain.

This is because the strain causes the complex structure of the bones at your back to get disturbed. If this pressure continues, the back can get permanently damaged.

Another reason which can cause your muscles and bones to get strained is slouching when you sit in chairs.

No matter how expensive your chair is, research has confirmed that if you regularly sit in a chair, you are likely to experience back pain. This is especially true if you sit for long hours without any breaks. This is because sitting for a long period of time reduces blood flow to you back, which can strain your muscles.

Also, it has been proven by research that sitting can be 30% more damaging for your back than standing or walking. Thus, in order to help prevent your back from serious damage, you need to walk around and do some activity regularly, especially if you spend much time sitting.

Weight gain and back pain?

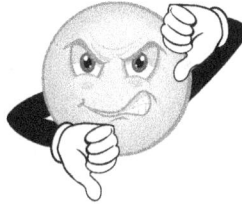

Being overweight can increase your chances of back pain by 20%.

If you live with a bulging belly, chances are higher that you may live with back pain too. It has been proven by research that weight gain is directly proportional to back pain. This means that as you gain weight, your chances of having back pain increases.

Weight gain comes with not just a bulging belly, but with the potential for lots of diseases as well. The reason why weight is such a big culprit is because of the strain it puts on different parts of our body, such as your heart and bones.

Extra pressure is also the reason for weight gain to be directly linked with back pain.

When you gain weight, you gain unnecessary calories. These calories are then turned into extra fat, and are stored in the body. This extra fat can put pressure on the muscles in the back, distorting the alignment of the bones. It is when the alignment is disturbed and the muscles are strained that you can experience pain.

Add to this the continuous slouching in a chair, and your pain can shoot up. If you are overweight, and your work involves sitting for a long period of time, there are very high chances of having strong back pain.

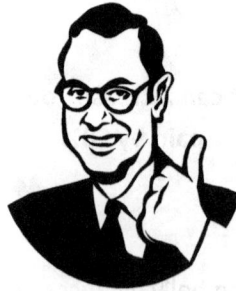

Reducing just 4 pounds can reduce 16% of your chances of back pain.

If extra fats and regular awkward postures continue working together, then you may permanently damage your back. It is best to try and fix both of these factors, but while it may not be easy for you to quit your job and look for a more comfortable one, it is probably easier to reduce your weight.

However, if you continue your life with a bulging belly, then your life may be negatively affected. Consider yourself in the middle of an important job, and imagine getting severe back pain. Will you be able to continue with your work? Maybe not.

The pain can sometimes be so severe that you cannot concentrate on anything else, except the pain itself.

Therefore, the next time you plan on eating junk food, imagine the pain you may experience if you gain weight and strain your back. While weight gain can cause many problems, weight loss can do the opposite. If you start losing your weight, you may significantly reduce your chances of a strained back.

Did you read the above statement? It says reducing a little weight can greatly decrease your chances of back pain. This has also been confirmed by research. Hence, weight loss has a lot of potential benefits, reduction in back pain being one of them.

When you consume fewer calories your muscles and bones will be under less stress and pressure.

This means that you may be able to move your back more freely, with additional flexibility. Your chances of getting back pain can significantly reduce. Your overall life may improve.

Reduce back pain through weight loss

Here are some simple tips for you to follow to help you reduce back pain and weight simultaneously.

Exercise

Exercise is perhaps the best way to burn off the extra fat stored in your body. Unless you burn off these extra fats, you may not be able to achieve significant results. Hence, it is important that you start an exercise regime to burn off the extra fat.

Research has also confirmed that following a good exercise regime can significantly lessen back pain. You should, however, be careful with the selection of exercises. If you suffer from severe back pain, do not over stress your muscles by exercising.

You should also select exercises which will be soothing for your back. Do not select harsh exercises as they may damage your back. You can perhaps do yoga, as yoga is also a very good tool to relieve you from back pain.

Aerobic exercise is another option. It has been confirmed by researchers that aerobic activity can reduce your weight and back pain. This is because aerobic activities are usually gentle in nature, and can help alleviate the problems in your back.

You can perhaps go out for cycling on a calm sunny morning, or can call your friends and go for a walk. If you do these exercises 5 days a week, then you are most likely to reap good results.

Your weight may significantly reduce, and the chances of getting back pain can lessen.

If your health does not permit you to exercise 5 times a week, start with lower amounts of exercise. Gradually, you may notice a boost in your stamina. You may then be able to exercise for longer periods of time.

Include exercise in your daily routine and you may very well experience the benefits of weight loss.

Diet

It is not just the exercise which can help you in reducing your weight and back pain. Your diet plays an important role too. You need to cut down the storage of extra fat in your body by reducing the number of calories that you eat.

If you gain more calories and burn less of them, the difference of the calories will be stored as extra fat. It is essential that you eat foods which are low in calories and high in essential nutrients.

You don't have to starve yourself to reduce weight. You just have to be wise enough to select foods with lower calories.

Eat fresh fruits and vegetables daily to aid your back with the strength it needs. Also, reduce your consumption of junk food, saturated and trans-fats, as they are damaging for your weight and back.

With patience and practice, you can see positive results. Hence, follow a good exercise regime, reduce your fats, and you should see your weight and back pain being reduced.

Chapter 22 – Stop Depression

We all face ups and downs and mood swings in life. These emotions are usually short lived, and vanish as time passes. However, depression brings pretty strong feelings of sadness, hopelessness and discouragement that can last for months or even longer.

Depression is a very serious illness. Many people suffering from it never seek treatment. However, the majority of people who seek treatment may overcome this problem.

Depression can have a very negative impact on your life. Hence, it is essential that you reduce your chances of getting depression. As you will shortly see, your weight loss regime can significantly help you in this regard.

There are four types of depression. Major depression is the strongest depression among all the four types.

It interferes with the person's ability to perform common activities, such as eating, sleeping and working. Some people may face this type of depression once in their life. However, most of the people suffering from it face it more than once in their lifetime.

Minor depression is a type of depression in which the person faces symptoms for about two weeks. However, if minor depression is not treated, it is can turn into major depression.

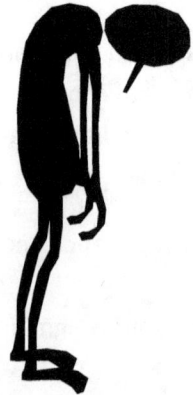

Signs of Depression

People suffering from depression can act, think or react in a different manner. It affects their way of thinking, and can cause physical symptoms such as body pain.

Negative Feelings: People facing depression may develop negative thinking and low mood. Being sad, discouraged and having the feeling of being defeated are among the many feelings in depression.

Someone with depression may also get annoyed, irritated and can get angry easily. Many depressive people feel guilty, unworthy and rejected. They often try to harm themselves because of the feeling of being unwanted and unworthy.

Low Motivation and Energy are also some of the signs of a depressive person. They may feel tired and lethargic most of the time. These people might also face trouble with motivation regarding a particular goal.

Social Withdrawal: One of the signs of depression is that the person avoids social interactions because of low energy and feeling of being unworthy and unwanted. The person may also feel difficulty in concentrating on one particular activity such as school, homework or office work.

Causes of Depression

Depression is caused by an imbalance of chemicals in the brain. These chemicals are the neurotransmitters that affect the mood of a person. There can be many other factors which cause this imbalance. Sometimes multiple factors affect a person and land him/her in a state of depression.

Inherited: Many people who suffer from depression usually have a close relative such as parents or siblings who suffer from this problem. This problem may run in the family, thus, other members of the family may have higher chances of facing depression.

Stressful Situation: Some people also get in a state of depression when they are not able to handle a stressful situation appropriately. The most common factor is financial problems, such as an inability to pay back a loan, which can trigger depression in the person.

Overweight: Being overweight is one of the major causes of depression in people. People may not feel good about their body and avoid social interactions. Feelings of being ugly can cause sadness in the person, especially in girls. If action is not taken, this sadness can last for a longer time and can increase the chances of major depression.

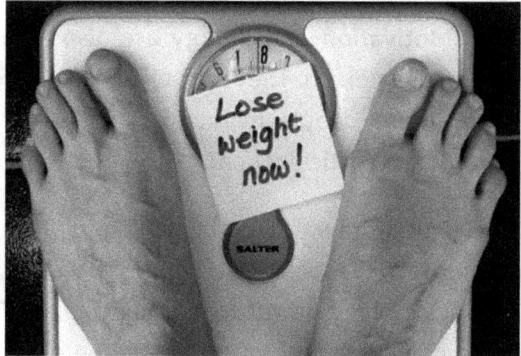

Hence, if you are among those who feel bad about their increasing weight, start taking steps to reduce the extra fat. This is because continuous bad feelings about your weight can land you into depression.

Poor Sleeping Habit: This is one of the most ignored causes of depression. However, it can lead to major depression if not taken care of. If a person does not sleep adequately, then the brain does not have time to renew its brain cells. The brain can stop functioning properly and this can lead to depression.

Depression can make your life miserable if it is not dealt with correctly. It is essential to identify the root cause of depression to overcome this problem.

One of the major causes of depression in people, especially women is being overweight.

If you are overweight, you may feel insecure because of your body. This can lead to avoidance of social interactions and trigger sadness. The feeling of being helpless and hopeless can start to prevail in your mind, which is a major cause of depression.

It can possibly cause major problems with your career as depression can lead to missing days of work and lack of concentration.

You can also face family issues. Depressive people tend to lock themselves in their rooms, get annoyed and irritated easily.

You can feel dizzy at work because of sleep deprivation.

Depression can affect your overall life negatively. But you can take measures to avoid this type of problem. If you are depressed because of being overweight then exercise daily, try to eat fewer calories and do all possible things to decrease your weight.

Treatment of Depression and Weight Loss

One of the treatments for depression is medication. You can visit a doctor or psychologist who you can discuss this option with. If you are not in favour of medication then you can focus on a natural treatment of depression.

Eat Healthy: Many people start overeating in depression. So, one of the main things to control in depression is to eat healthy.

When you lose weight, your diet revolves around healthy fruits and vegetables. You also eat foods which are high in nutrients and low in calories. These are the foods which can reduce your chances of getting depression.

These foods make you feel fresh and healthy; hence you are probably less concerned about your weight. When you are not as concerned about your look and weight, you may not feel depressed. Also, with continuous practice of such a diet, you may start losing weight gradually.

You can choose healthy foods with low fats, as they can help you in losing weight. Moreover, foods with omega-3 and folic acids such as salmon and spinach can also help reduce depression.

Avoid foods that contain high sugar, such as sweets and soft drinks. When depressed, people tend to eat more junk food and desserts to feel better. But high sugar content can result in a glucose crash which has a depressing mood effect. Avoiding sugar can help you to lose weight, which can then help in overcoming a depressive state.

Exercise: You may not know this, but exercise is an anti-depressant. When you follow a good exercise regime to help reduce your weight, the depression may also reduce.

Exercise releases certain chemicals in the body, which can make you feel fresh and healthy. Also, exercise is a very good tool to burn the extra fat around your bellies. When you see your bellies and bodies getting back into shape, you may not feel depressed about yourself.

Even if you have a family history of depression, feeling good about yourself through exercise is a very good tool to reduce your chances of getting depression.

Apart from exercises, you should also continue activities that you love such as yoga, swimming etc. This can help you to feel better about yourself and gives a sense of direction in your life.

Set goals during your exercise regime. Start by aiming to reduce a few pounds in a month. This gives your life a sense of direction and motivates you when you are down. As you set and achieve goals in your life, you may feel better about yourself.

Adequate sleep: It will be difficult for you to lose weight if you do not sleep well. Same is the case with depression. As you have read above, inadequate sleep can also trigger depression.

If you are following a good weight loss regime, you are more likely to sleep well.

This can give enough time for your brain to renew its cells, which is important for its proper functioning. This can also improve your daily routine, reducing the chances of depression.

Your weight loss regime can help decrease the signs of depression. Try to sleep at least 8 hours a day, and try to sleep and wake up at a set time.

To conclude, depression is a dangerous disease which should be avoided. It can jeopardize your whole life if you do not try and take measures to reduce the signs and symptoms. One of the major causes of depression is being overweight.

Reducing your weight can help decrease depressive feelings. Start by exercising daily and eating healthy foods.

Do you constantly feel low and tired? Do you often lack the energy and motivation to complete your work? If yes, then you have landed on the right chapter. We are going to tell you how your weight is directly linked to your energy levels.

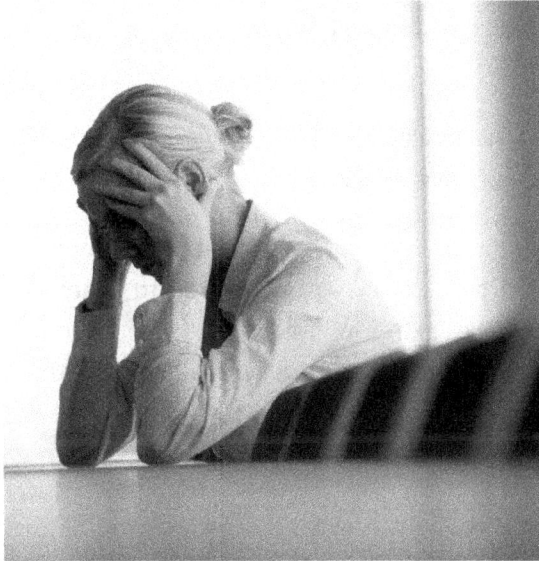

Fatigue and lack of energy is a very common problem. It is reported that at one point in time, around 10% of people feel tired and fatigued.

This lack of energy is usually not a serious issue and can be removed easily. However, if the problem persists, and you cannot concentrate on anything, then you should probably visit a doctor.

There can be many causes of lack of energy. Sometimes you may feel tired because of a medical illness. While in many cases issues with your lifestyle is the main reason for your lack of energy and motivation.

You may also feel tired and lazy all day if you do not get an adequate supply of water. If you do not drink at least 8 glasses of water a day, your body will not be able to function properly. Since water is required by every part of the body, your body parts will not perform well without enough water, potentially making you feel tired.

Sometimes the fatigue can be a serious symptom of a disease. One such example is anaemia.

Deficiency of iron is one of the most important medical reasons for fatigue. Iron deficiency can lead you to anaemia, which in turn can cause extreme fatigue. Hence, if you feel tired regularly, then you should visit your doctor, as this can be a symptom of anaemia.

Weight gain and lack of energy

Perhaps the most important culprit for your tiredness is your weight. If you suffer from the problem of being overweight, then you may also suffer from the problem of feeling tired all the time.

The reason why you gain weight is most likely because you consume unnecessary calories. These unnecessary calories are often stored in your body as fat, and are not burned off. Since fat is not being burned off to create energy for your body, you may feel tired.

Also, you can gain weight when you are inactive. When your life mostly revolves around inactivity and laziness, you do not burn proteins and carbohydrates. Proteins, carbohydrates and fats are the sources of energy for your body.

Your body produces energy when these nutrients are burnt. Since these nutrients are not being burnt in your inactive life, you may feel tired and lazy all day.

It has been proven through various researches that people who do not exercise feel much more tired as compared to people who do.

You also gain weight when you eat lots of sugary foods and chocolates. These sugary foods are high in bad sugar and low in essential nutrients, and are bad for your weight.

When you consume these foods you get a temporary burst of energy. The energy, however, wears off quickly, leaving you even more tired and fatigued. Hence, eating sugary foods can increase your weight, and can make you tired.

In some cases, weight gain may disturb a person to an extent that he or she may skip meals completely. This is a dangerous practice to follow. You should never skip meals, as skipping meals may completely deprive you of the energy you need.

Without energy, you may not be able to function well in your life. Be it your job or your home, constant tiredness may not let your work efficiently. You may want to go to bed or lounge on the couch, which may negatively affect your work.

Since lack of exercise and lack of a healthy diet may make you more tired, exercise and healthy diet may do the opposite. Reducing your weight may make you more active and motivated.

Exercise and energy

Exercise increases the power of your blood to carry oxygen to various parts of your body. This results in an increased capability of your cells to convert nutrients into energy.

When you exercise, your cells produce even greater levels of energy, helping to keep you active throughout the day.

You do not have to follow tough exercise regimes to increase your energy levels though. Even simple ones would do the job efficiently.

You may be surprised to know this, but research has shown that exercise can also train your DNA to work more efficiently. When you exercise and produce more energy, your DNA gets trained in the process, and your cells will naturally produce more energy. The more you exercise the more energy your body produces.

With busy schedules and tiredness, you may not feel like exercising. But, here we have very simple exercises for you which may not only reduce your weight, but may fill you up with energy.

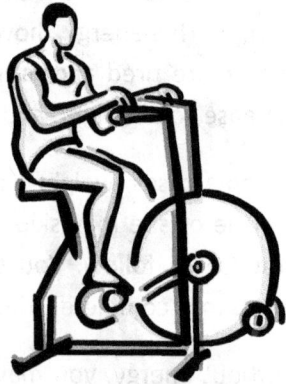

Walking

Walking is one of the easiest sources to reduce your weight, and to fill you up with energy. It reduces your weight by burning off the extra calories and fat. While doing so, it increases your heart beat, and the ability of your body to carry oxygen to different parts of the body.

It is when the oxygen is carried properly to the cells that the cells burn the nutrients to fill you up with energy. The more you walk, the more your body will keep you active.

Start your day with brisk walking. Get up a little early, call your friends, go out for a walk, and get an energetic start to your day.

Hopping and Skipping

Hopping is a great tool to reduce your weight, and to increase your energy. Hopping is a convenient exercise too. If you are one of those who do not get adequate time for exercises, then you should definitely consider hopping.

For hopping, you do not need to go out in a park, or to a gym. You can easily hop anywhere in your office or at home. It may seem silly if you hop in front of everyone in the office. Try and hop in some secluded space, and fill yourself with energy.

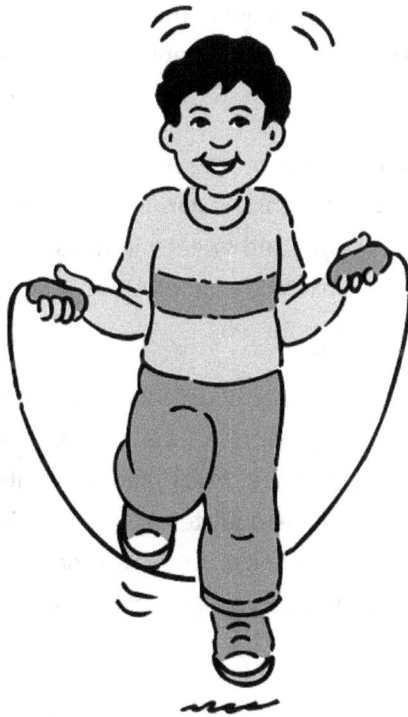

Hopping can fill you up with instant energy. It utilizes your whole body, keeping each and every part active. This can burn off the extra calories, keeping you active throughout the day.

Weight loss diet and energy

When you plan on losing weight, you should have planned to eat a healthy and balanced diet. This is because without a healthy diet, you may not be able to reduce your weight. This healthy diet is essential; as it can help you increase your energy.

Your diet should mostly consist of fruits and vegetables. Fruits and vegetables are very effective when it comes to weight loss and energy boost. The vitamins and minerals found in most of the fruits and vegetables can fill you up with ample amounts of energy.

Also, some of the fruits are filled with sugar and glucose. However, this sugar is different from the sugars found in chocolates and sweets, in the sense that they do not harm your body. Instead, they give you less calories, and more energy to perform your jobs.

For an energy boost you should also try foods with iron, as an iron deficiency can be a reason for being tired on a regular basis. Besides fruits and vegetables, your diet should also consist of lean proteins, whole grains and unsaturated fats. This is because these foods will not just help reduce your weight; they can give you an instant energy boost.

Tiredness and fatigue are very common problems which need to be dealt with. Since most of the time weight gain is a cause of fatigue, one should plan on reducing weight.

Section 3

The Extras

Recall the story we told you in the first two introductions about Edward. He was a business man who started his own business with much enthusiasm. With a growing and expanding business, he became rich and successful.

There was however a time when Edward's obesity interfered with his life and business. He lost his health and wealth. He went into depression and could no longer manage his business.

However, after realizing that weight gain was the cause of his problems, he worked hard to regain his previous shape. He managed his diet and regularly followed an exercise regime.

As his weight was being reduced, positive things started happening in his life. He was able to control his blood pressure and his depression. He became more active, and his brain was now able to concentrate on his lost business.

As you might have read earlier, weight loss comes with a lot of benefits for a person. Like Edward, who regained his lost life, you can gain it back too if weight has affected you.

Weight loss can give you a slim and healthy figure to pose with. In fact, weight loss has many long term benefits on your health.

Weight loss, while a challenge, is a worthy goal. By practicing the tips mentioned in the previous two sections, you should see your weight reducing. There are however, many other extra things which you need to know while you reduce your weight.

The first section of the book was designed to give you a good idea about how to reduce your weight.

The second section then continued to tell you the additional benefits which you can gain once your weight is under control.

Now, the third section will increase your knowledge and will tell you all the essential things which you need to know besides a healthy diet and healthy exercises.

This section will first focus on all the foods which you should incorporate in your daily lives. These are the essential foods which will help you reduce your weight. Next, we will tell you all the foods which should be avoided by you, so that you can live a healthy lifestyle.

This section will also focus on calculating your Body Mass Index (BMI) and your weight category. With this you will be able to set a target weight and work effectively towards it. This section will also give you a brief idea of the exercises which you should do to burn the extra calories.

This last section of the book will enhance your knowledge about healthy weight loss. If you want to effectively reduce your weight, and see your body coming back into shape, then you should read and follow this section.

Chapter 24 – Foods to Enjoy

Foods that you eat determine whether you will gain weight or lose it. It is essential to choose your food plan carefully when you are on a mission to lose weight.

The formula of gaining or losing weight is very simple. If you eat more calories than you burn, you will end up gaining weight. On the other hand, if you burn more calories than you eat, you can achieve your goal of losing weight.

Crafting your diet plan carefully does not mean that you end up eating foods that are miserable in taste. If you do so, you might not be able to continue with your mission of losing weight for too long. Choose foods that are good in taste and can help you in losing weight.

Below are some of the foods which you can enjoy without having to worry about gaining weight.

Increase your intake of vitamin C

Vitamin C is well known for fighting colds and improving skin. However, few people know that vitamin C is actually very helpful when it comes to weight loss. Vitamin C is a fat burner and increasing its intake can help you reduce fat.

Men are advised to consume at least 90 milligrams of vitamin C daily, whereas women are advised to consume 70 milligrams.

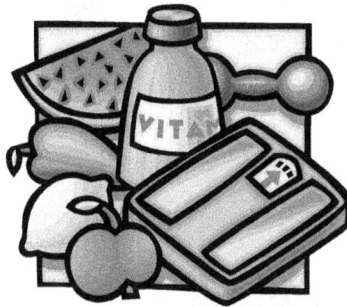

Fruits with high levels of vitamin C are **papaya** with 188 mg of vitamin C, **bell pepper** with 117 mg in 1 raw cup and **strawberries** with 85 mg of vitamin C in a serving of 1 cup.

Apart from foods with vitamin C there are many other foods which are helpful when it comes to weight loss. If you stick to these foods, you should be able to achieve your set target weight.

Oats:

Oats contain high amounts of fiber, so they will make you feel full throughout the day. Only a half cup of oats contains 4.6g of resistant starch. This is a very useful carbohydrate as it fastens your metabolism and can help your body in burning fat.

Salmon:

Many people do not know that eating salmon can actually help them in losing weight. Salmon contains monounsaturated fatty acids (MUFA). MUFA is a healthy unsaturated fat. This is helpful when it comes to weight loss. According to a study, people consuming MUFA lost an average of 9 pounds whereas people who lacked MUFA in their diet gained about 6 pounds of weight on average.

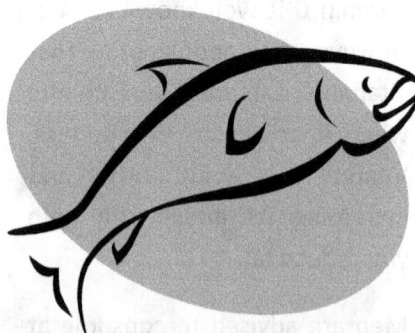

Pears:

This fruit is packed with 15% of your daily fiber need. According to a study, women who ate about 3 pears per day consumed fewer calories than the women who didn't. They also lost weight at a faster rate than the women who did not consume pears. You should not peel the skin, as it is the skin where most of the fiber is stored.

Grapefruit:

If you cannot alter your diet, then eating just a half grapefruit before each meal can actually help you lose about 1 pound each week. One of the compounds in this fruit lowers your insulin, a hormone that stores fat in your body. This can lead to rapid weight loss. Moreover, it contains 90% percent of water. This can help you feel full.

Eggs:

They have a bad reputation when it comes to weight loss. However, it can surprise you that eating eggs for breakfast instead of bagels will help you lose weight. An egg is loaded with proteins; hence, eating it for breakfast can lower your appetite for the rest of the day.

According to a study, women who eat eggs for their breakfast lose twice as much weight than women who started their day by eating bagels.

Dark Chocolate:

Are you surprised to see dark chocolate written here in this chapter? We are sure this will make chocolate lovers happy.

Dark chocolate contains monounsaturated fatty acids (MUFA) that boosts metabolism of your body. This can result in burning of fat. So, chocolate lovers can stop worrying, as eating dark chocolate can help them in losing weight.

Cheese:

People also avoid cheese when they are trying to lose weight. However, feta and goat cheese contain healthy fatty acids that can help you reduce belly fat. Look for "grass fed" cheese that contains the highest amount of this healthy fatty acid.

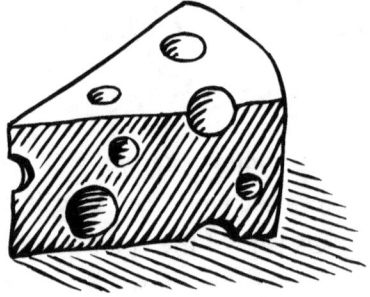

Foods which make you feel full

Milk:

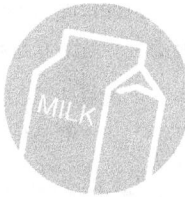

> **Drink milk for breakfast to reduce your appetite for the whole day.**

Milk is well known for its supply of calcium. However, few people know that it helps you control your hunger as well. People who drink milk daily are reported to have less body fat and a controlled appetite. So, milk can play an essential part when it comes to weight loss. It does not only assist you in weight loss, but can also provide your body with necessary calcium.

Avocados:

Avocados can prove to be helpful when it comes to weight loss. This is because they contain a healthy acid known as oleic acid which helps in weight loss. They can actually help your body to reduce the hunger and melt away the fat in your body. Apart from good fats and acids, avocados are also packed with proteins and fiber which further helps your body to feel full.

Brown Rice:

It is one of the friendly foods when it comes to weight loss. Only half a cup of brown rice contains 1.7 g of resistant starch that burns fat in your body and increases your metabolism. Moreover, brown rice is filling and heavy but low in calories.

According to a study, women who ate white rice gained 6 times more weight over a period of six years than women who ate brown rice.

When you are on a weight loss mission, try to choose foods very carefully. This is because some foods that are known to increase body fat actually decrease fat in your body.

For breakfast, try to consume food which helps you feel full throughout the day. In this way, you may eat less and can more easily lose weight just by carefully choosing your food.

You should, however, never avoid foods which provide necessary nutrients to your body and are essential for a healthy body. You should remember that losing weight does not mean making your body weak and malnourished. Enjoy the foods mentioned above, and cherish a healthy weight.

Chapter 25 – Foods to Avoid

Foods can turn into added weight or they can help you lose weight. It all depends on the foods you eat, and the time and quantity of those foods. If you are planning on losing weight, then read this chapter and find out which foods are bad for your weight.

A quick reminder

A diet based on 2,000 calories per day should have no more than 66 grams of fat, less than 20 grams of saturated fats, no more than 2,400 milligrams of sodium and 300 grams of total carbohydrates, including sugars.

Carefully craft your diet plan so that you do not eat foods that add to the fat in your body. Also, avoid foods with high calories as they can result in consumption of calories more than your body can burn. This can result in weight gain.

Foods with high calories

In order to lose weight, you should avoid eating foods that supply large amount of calories to your body.

Margarine contains high amount of trans fats. This can lower good cholesterol in your body and increase bad cholesterol levels. One tablespoon of margarine contains about 100 calories.

Soda contains high level of sugar content. Almost the calories provided by soda come from sugar. It can also be called liquid candy. Such high amounts of sugar consumption are responsible for fuelling obesity in people. Apart from calories, it also causes tooth decay and weakens your bones. This can result in a weak body if you continue to consume it.

Bagels are considered to be weight loss friendly by many people. But you will be surprised to learn that bagels can actually result in weight gain. Calories in one bagel are equivalent to 4-5 slices of white bread.

Hot Dogs contain high amounts of saturated fats. 80 percent of calories in hot dogs come from unsaturated fats. These unsaturated fats can keep on adding to your belly fat.

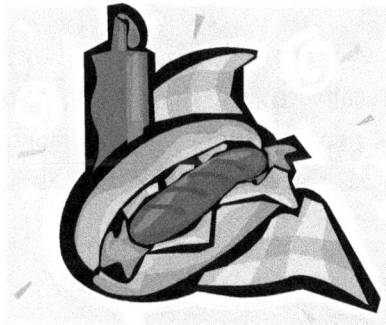

Movie Theatre Popcorns contain very high amount of calories and fats. They can contain about 1,200 calories as they are normally prepared with coconut oil and butter. Moreover, topping adds more fat and calories to this snack. Fats and calories in these popcorns are equivalent to three large sized fast food burgers. The next time you plan on going to the movies, make sure you eat some healthy snack, instead of high calorie popcorn.

Pizzas with thick and dense crust can actually shock your body with 1,300 calories. It can also contain high amounts of saturated fats, storing more fat in your body. You may like pizza a lot, but in order to reduce your weight, you should consume less pizza.

Peanut Butter contains high amount of calories and carbohydrates. One tablespoon of peanut butter adds an average of 192 calories to your meal. Thus, peanut butter too should not be a major part of your diet.

Chocolate Spread is packed with high amount of calories and sugar content. Just 100 grams of chocolate nut spread stores up to 540 calories. You may love eating bread slices with chocolate spread on them. But, in order to reduce your weight, you should let go off this food.

White Rice adds very little nutritional value to the body. Being high in calories, it can also spike the sugar level in the body. This is dangerous for people suffering from diabetes. You should choose brown rice instead of white rice as it can help you reduce your weight.

Diet Sodas contain chemically prepared sweeteners. Apart from adding calories to your body, it also raises many issues regarding health in your body.

Foods to avoid at breakfast

It is very important to eat a healthy and balanced breakfast. If you eat a breakfast that is low in calories and saturated fats, you should have an energetic start to your day. This can help you feel full all day long thus, you may eat less.

This can play a major role in decreasing or maintaining weight.

Many people eat unhealthy and high calorie breakfasts. This bulks up fat in their body. You should try to avoid eating these foods in your breakfast to lose your weight and stay away from the fat.

Sugary cereals

Cereals that contain high amount of sugar can actually result in increasing weight. These cereals are usually packed with high amount of calories and carbohydrates. This lowers your metabolism so your body burns fat and carbs slower than usual. All these factors can result in an increase in your weight.

Packaged pancakes

Packaged pancakes that contain artificial maple syrup are actually risky for your health. Corn syrup with high fructose content can result in visceral fat and abdominal obesity. This can possibly result in more fat in your body and high sugar levels. This can decrease your energy level in the middle of the day.

Foods to avoid in Lunch

Meals you eat at lunch are supposed to increase your energy levels for the rest of the day, not your weight for the rest of your life.

There are certain foods which you should try to avoid at lunch to avoid weight gain.

Hamburger

While you are working in your office or busy at your home, you may not get enough time to prepare a healthy lunch for yourself. This is why many people opt for fast foods, and quite often hamburger, which is one of the most common foods at lunch.

Hamburger is usually accompanied by fries, bacon and a supersized bun. This increases the amount of calories in the hamburger. Moreover, fries contain trans fats, which are categorized as unhealthy fats and can result in increasing weight. In the middle of the day it is unadvisable to eat excess calories as it can result in low energy levels.

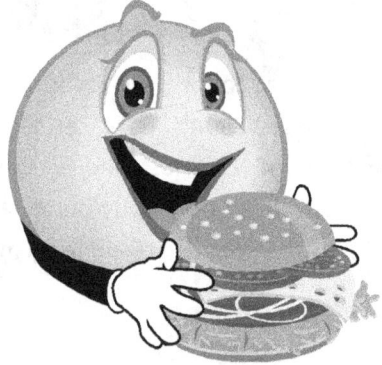

Premade sandwiches

Almost every store provides premade sandwiches to its customers for their convenience. Without a doubt, they are convenient as they save time of preparing a fresh sandwich. But on the other hand, they store high amounts of calories and unhealthy fats. They feel light to eat but requires a heavy workout to burn its unhealthy fat.

Foods to avoid at dinner

It is advisable to eat food that makes your stomach no more than half full at dinner. Avoid foods with high trans and saturated fats. As there is usually very little activity at night the body can bulk up on unhealthy fats instead of burning them.

If you avoid foods which contain high amount of calories, carbohydrates, trans fats and saturated fats, you may see a significant reduction in your weight. Follow the guidance we have given you here, and start working to get your desired shape back.

Coffee is perhaps one of the most popular drinks in the world. It is one of the oldest and readily available drugs on the market. There are many negative things about coffee but also good things at the same time. There is a lot of misinformation about coffee and its effects.

Some Facts about Coffee

- ► Caffeine occurs naturally in more than 60 plants including coffee beans and tea leaves.
- ► It is sometimes added to foods, drinks, and medicines.
- ► Ninety percent of people in the world use caffeine in one form or another.
- ► Whether caffeine is consumed in food or as a medicine, it alters the way your brain and body work, changing how you behave and feel.

Caffeine is known to stimulate your central nervous system.

It is a well-known fact that drinking more coffee can actually improve the workings of your brain, and your nerves. Coffee can make these parts more active and energetic. You will notice that drinking a cup of coffee can make your brain more alert too. You should not over-consume it though.

Caffeine makes you more physically active.

Caffeine, the main ingredient in coffee, acts as a stimulant to the central nervous system. This is why an individual feels energized when he or she has coffee.

Coffee can also help you overcome constipation.

Research suggests that coffee has a simulative effect on the colon. However, coffee may result in loose bowel movements as well. Hence, make sure you do not over-consume it.

Drinking coffee can aid in achieving an ideal weight.

Studies suggest that caffeine leads to a temporary increase in the metabolic rate and the rate of breakdown of fat. Therefore, people trying to lose weight can benefit by increasing their coffee consumption. It has also been suggested that coffee helps you exercise due to its ability to energize.

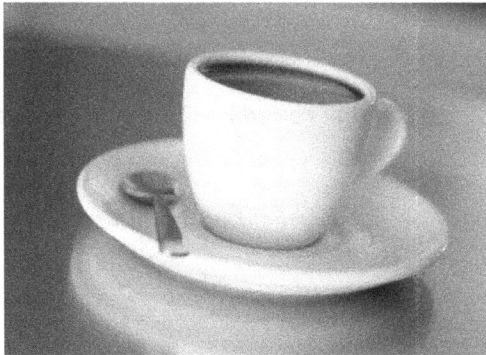

Coffee can also be beneficial to a person's health.

According to researchers coffee drinkers are less likely to develop diabetes, Parkinson's disease or liver cirrhosis. There is also evidence that coffee can help prevent cavities, cure headaches and even lift moods. However, coffee is not good for pregnant women. This is primarily because coffee may affect the baby adversely by impacting the baby's heartbeat.

Drinking coffee also affects the memory temporal lobe as well as the attention-controlling part of the brain.

This suggests that coffee may temporarily enhance your memory and attention. It has also been observed that people who drink a moderate amount of coffee are less likely to develop Alzheimer's or dementia in old age.

Reduction in breast size

Research suggests that women who drink three or more cups of coffee a day might observe a reduction in the size of their breasts. But caffeine helps boost fertility in men. According to researchers caffeine has a positive effect on sperm motility- which is the process in which the sperm fertilizes the egg and so could increase the chances of getting pregnant.

The best time to drink coffee is NOT when you wake up.

Coffee impacts Cortisol (a stress hormone) which is already high when you wake up. Cortisol affects the alertness of the body and it generally peaks during 8 and 9 am. Therefore, the first cup of coffee should be taken during 9-11 am.

Coffee takes around 4 and 6 hours to break down inside your body and so it should not be taken before bedtime. It might take you longer to go to sleep, which in turn might adversely affect your daily routine.

Some harmful effects of coffee

While it may appear that coffee has many favorable outcomes drinking it can lead to several adverse effects. Drinking coffee can irritate the lining of the small intestine, potentially leading to abdominal spasms and cramps. Sometimes it may also lead to heartburns, as compounds in coffee such as decaf can contribute to acid reflux problems.

Heavy coffee drinkers may have difficulty in getting minerals in their diets. This is because coffee affects the ability of the stomach to absorb iron, leading to irregularities in bowel movements.

A large consumption of coffee can **increase stress and tension** in an individual primarily because of the release of stress hormones such as epinephrine and norepinephrine. These chemicals increase the body's heart rate, blood pressure and tension levels. We often say we need to drink coffee to give us energy. But for many of us, it has gone beyond energy and turned into a stressful situation which makes it difficult to relax.

Each person has a different level of tolerance for caffeine and sometimes a **caffeine overdose** might occur. While it is rare, it can lead to many adverse symptoms including death. People allergic to caffeine suffer from reactions such as hives and pain. Although not a true allergy, many report very negative symptoms after consuming even the smallest amounts.

> **Experts agree that four to seven cups of coffee or more each day is too much.**

Caffeine speeds up the urination cycle, but "steals" calcium which is lost through urine. Long term, heavy caffeine use can lead to a rapid development of osteoporosis. However caffeine may reduce the risk of skin cancer. Also, if coffee is combined with exercise, the risks of sun induced skin cancer are greatly reduced. It has even been suggested that caffeine reduces post gym muscle pain.

Some studies show that caffeine causes a physical dependence or addiction. If you are addicted to coffee, chances are that you may feel bad when you stop drinking coffee. You may feel depressed and irritable all the time. Also, you may experience physical pains, such as muscles aches and headaches.

> **Ideal coffee intake:**
>
> **Doctors suggest 100 to 200 mg should be the limit of intake per day.**

The list of caffeine's potential benefits is interesting. Any regular coffee drinker may tell you that caffeine improves alertness, concentration, energy, clear-headedness, and feelings of sociability. Even scientific studies support these subjective findings. Therefore, caffeine can have favorable effects on an individual if taken in the right amount and at the right time.

Do you realize that one of the main culprits of your weight gain is the extra fat stored in your body? You gain weight when your calorie input is greater than your calorie output. The difference of the calories is then stored in your body as body fat.

This body fat can be extremely troublesome. The excess fat stored in your body can also make you suffer from various diseases. One of the diseases that you may get is high blood pressure.

You get high blood pressure when the excess fat disturbs the flow of blood. The fat may block your nerves in some cases, and they may burst. This excess fat can damage your heart, and hence, should be controlled.

Apart from high blood pressure, you may get a lot of other diseases because of your weight and fat. In order to effectively reduce your weight, you need to cut down your fats.

But, how do you calculate the amount of fat stored in your body? Here we have a very simple tool for you to use to calculate the amount of fat stored.

Body mass index (BMI) is a measure for the human body. It uses height and weight of a human body to give the estimate of fat present in the body.

BMI can be a good measure to know the risk of health problems. The higher the BMI, the higher the risk of facing health issues.

High BMI can indicate the risk of certain health issues such as certain cancers, high blood pressure and heart attacks. In order to prevent yourself from various diseases, you should learn how to calculate your BMI.

It also indicates whether you are healthy, underweight or overweight. This helps you decide whether to lose weight or to gain weight depending upon the ratio of your body's height and weight.

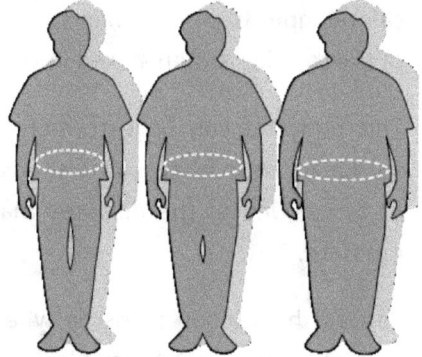

How to calculate BMI

You can calculate your BMI either manually or by using BMI calculators. However, calculating BMI manually can give more accurate data than BMI calculators. By calculating manually, you will use actual measurements of your body weight and height.

Follow these steps to calculate BMI manually:

Step 1

Measuring weight is the key ingredient of BMI. Measure the weight of your body using a good bathroom scale. Note down your weight in pounds. The most suitable time to measure your weight is right after you wake up.

You should avoid measuring weight right after you eat food. This is because you may temporary gain weight right after you eat.

Step 2

208

After weight, **calculating your height** is the thing you need to do. Measure your height in inches. To measure your height accurately, you can stand straight against the wall with your head held straight. Mark your height using a pencil. Then use a yard stick, or measuring tape, to measure the distance between the floor and your placed mark. This distance will be your height.

Just in case you are not sure about the accuracy of your height, get a friend to measure your height for you. The height measured by your friend, or a relative, will be much more accurate.

Step 3

Take a **square of your height** in inches. Or simply multiply the number with the same number once.

For example, you measured your height at 70 inches. Multiply it by 70 once (70x70). Or, simply take the square of the number $(70)^2$. $(70)^2 = 4,900$

Step 4

The fourth step is to **divide your weight by the square of your height** that you calculated in step 3. For example, suppose you calculated your weight to be 180 pounds. Divide 180 by the square of 70 (4,900) you calculated in the previous step.

> **Step 4: Weight (in pounds) divided by square of height**
>
> **180 / 4,900 = 0.0367346**

Now multiply **the answer of step 4 by 703** which is a conversion number. Skip this step if you used kilograms and meters to measure your weight and height.

> **Step 5: Step 4 x 703**
>
> **0.0367346 x 703 = 25.82**

How to read BMI

Are you feeling confused with so many numbers and calculations? You need not worry, because we are here to tell you what this calculation actually meant.

The final result of your BMI calculation will tell whether you have excess weight, normal weight or you are under weight. Follow these guidelines to see in which category you belong to:

- ▶ If your BMI score is below 18.5, it means you are underweight and you should gain weight to avoid health issues.
- ▶ BMI score that lies between 18.5 and 24.9 means that you have ideal weight.
- ▶ BMI score of 25.0 – 29.9 means that you are overweight and you should lose some weight to live a healthy life.
- ▶ And BMI score of 30.0 plus means that you are obese and should consult a doctor regarding your weight.

In our example, the calculated BMI was 25.82, which according to the guideline above, means that the person is overweight. The person should work towards reducing his weight. This can then promote him to the category of healthy weight.

While calculating your BMI, however, make sure you take accurate measurements. This is because inaccuracy can lead to wrong results.

For example, if you miscalculate your weight, then you may end up being in the healthy category, while you actually are overweight. This may make you feel satisfied about your health. With a misconception of being healthy, you may continue with your unhealthy eating habits. This can then lead to serious health issues.

To conclude, BMI is a great tool to see how much weight you have gained because of the extra fat. If you belong to the category of overweight, or obese, then that means that you have excess fat stored in your body. The excess fat is not being burnt off, and is increasing your weight.

You should, therefore, set a desired weight target to promote yourself to the healthy category. Start exercising to burn the calories and fat. Also, make sure you avoid all the foods which are likely to fill you up with extra calories.

Chapter 28 – Do's and Don'ts for a Healthy Lifestyle

We've all probably heard the saying 'A healthy life is a happy life.' Living a healthy life cannot only make you feel better and happy today, it can also help you avoid a variety of health problems in old age. By simply making some positive changes today, we may avoid problems in the future.

Do's	
Sleep well	An average adult needs 7-9 hours of sleep in order to function well in daily life. If you are constantly missing out on sleep, you may experience serious effects physically as well as psychologically. Sleep helps to improve an individual's memory, creativity and alertness to face the challenges of everyday life.
Drink plenty of water	The human body is comprised of approximately 60 percent water. While it is been a matter of dispute as to how much water the body actually needs, its necessity in the lives of humans is self-evident. We constantly excrete water throughout the day due to normal bodily functions and therefore, we must replenish that water. However, that does not mean that you must hydrate yourself with sodas. You should avoid such cravings. The added bonus about drinking water is that it can help you reduce weight.
Move your body	Do not make excuses for sitting at a desk all day

	and on the couch all evening. You cannot get healthy if you live an inactive life. You should regularly go out for a walk, and exercise. For simple shopping, prefer walking to the nearby store, instead of driving. The next time you need to get something from a retail store ditch your car and walk.

You should also take a break during the workday for a quick walk or a stretch at your desk. It's been shown that simple activities like taking a walk around the office or even bending down to tie your shoelaces will vary your heart rate. It can also burn a certain amount of calories. |
| **Exercise** | Going to a gym may seem like a chore but once you exert the initial effort you may soon realize that it is worth the pain. Start and finish your workout with stretching. Go to the gym 4 to 5 days a week so that your body adapts much quickly. However exercise in moderation in order to avoid injuries.

If going to the gym is not possible there are several alternatives which you can take up to stay fit. Gardening, housekeeping and even walking a few miles can help your body.

If you have problems in getting motivated, call your friends. Ask them to join in with you or motivate you. Or join a group or club where other people are also looking for healthy weight loss solutions. Discuss new ways of getting healthy. This can help to motivate you to work |

	hard and reduce your weight.
Track your progress	Know what you weigh. Being overweight and being underweight are not healthy states of being. Find out your ideal weight either by visiting your doctor, or by referring to a weight chart. However, that is just the beginning. Once you start working on your body you should track your progress with a fitness and/or diet journal. This can help you track your habits and help you to change the bad ones.
Eat healthy food	Choose food that contains minimal amounts of unhealthy fats. Unhealthy fats include both trans fats and saturated fats. These fats can raise your cholesterol level, which in turn might result in increased risk for heart disease. Eat more real, fresh food in the form of fruits and vegetables. You should also avoid processed foods. This is because processed foods are loaded with ingredients which may be harmful and are not good for your health and weight. In addition to that, keep sugar under scrutiny. This is because if sugar is taken in large amounts, it may result in obesity. Additionally, doctors have started prescribing better nutrition as a way to remind patients how important it is for their health. Use your willpower when you go grocery

	shopping and stock your house with healthy fruit and vegetables. When your refrigerator is filled with healthy foods, you are less likely to eat junk food. Even if you crave for sugars and saturated fats, not keeping them in your house can reduce your temptations.
Don'ts	
Don't: Skip breakfast.	The first meal of the day does not only refresh the human body and mind; it also plays an important role in a person's healthy lifestyle. It has been shown that kids score better on tests and in school after eating breakfast. Opt for 300-500 calories including proteins and include fruits and vegetables in your diet.
Don't: spend time with negative people.	We all know someone who will consistently point to the negative. Spending a lot of time with such a person may eventually get you down as well; it's almost impossible to ignore the negativity. Stay positive and remind yourself about the good things in life. You might feel guilty about walking away, but your mood and outlook for the rest of the day will be much better.
Don't: Eat midnight snacks.	No more late night eating. You should not eat snacks after 6:30 pm, as they are likely to increase your weight. If you are really hungry in the middle of the night, you can always eat

	fruits and healthy snacks.
Don't: Overeat at a meal.	Eating massive amounts of food at breakfast, lunch or dinner is not the wisest idea. Eat more frequent, smaller meals or snacks throughout the day, and you shouldn't be starving when mealtime comes around. This way your digestive system should function more adequately.
Don't: Go to extremes.	Remember that you should never overdo anything when it comes to your health. Implement a diet and exercise regimen you can stick with for the long run. Make a long term commitment but set your goals realistically

Follow these simple guidelines, and you should see your weight being reduced. You should not just get back a slim physique; you should feel healthy and active throughout the day. You should be able to live a healthy lifestyle if you follow the 'Do's' and avoid the 'Don'ts'.

Chapter 29 – Get Active

As kids most of us loved being active on the playground. It just came naturally. We loved moving around and running and staying fit. However, as we get older we realize that the responsibilities of everyday life can be so exhausting that we hardly have time to stay active.

Why is there a need to be active?

You should realise that you gain weight when you consume a lot of calories but do not burn them off properly. Therefore, in order to reduce your weight, you usually limit your intake of calories. However, in order to reduce weight, it is equally important that you burn off those calories by staying active.

Without activity, these calories can be stored as fat in your body. This extra fat can lead you to many diseases. Therefore, staying active is a great tool to keep those extra calories and diseases at bay.

Without regular activity, the body organs can begin to deteriorate and lose their ability to function adequately. Physical activity is beneficial to both the mental as well as physical state. It can help avoid serious problems such as obesity, heart diseases and even cancer.

Physical activity contributes to the overall positive well-being of an individual. The leading cause of some serious diseases such as diabetes and obesity are associated with an inactive life style.

Being physically active has a number of advantages. It increases your chances of living longer, and can make you feel better about yourself. It decreases the chance of becoming depressed and even helps you achieve a healthy weight and maintain it. You can also develop a better outlook on life with exercise.

As we become older our metabolism slows down. Therefore, in order to maintain an energy balance we should move more and eat less. Staying active even helps us move around more efficiently.

How to stay active?

Exercising is perhaps the best way to stay active.

Studies suggest that for each hour of exercise you do you gain about two hours of life expectancy. Even moderate exercise such as brisk walking has its benefits.

Exercising improves blood circulation, and helps keep weight under control. It improves blood cholesterol levels and even helps prevent and manages high blood pressure. It has also been observed that exercising helps manage stress, release tension, and promotes enthusiasm and optimism.

In children, it helps to establish good heart-healthy habits and counters the conditions that lead to heart attack and stroke later in life. Whereas in older people, exercising can help prevent chronic illnesses and diseases associated with aging and maintains quality of life and independence longer.

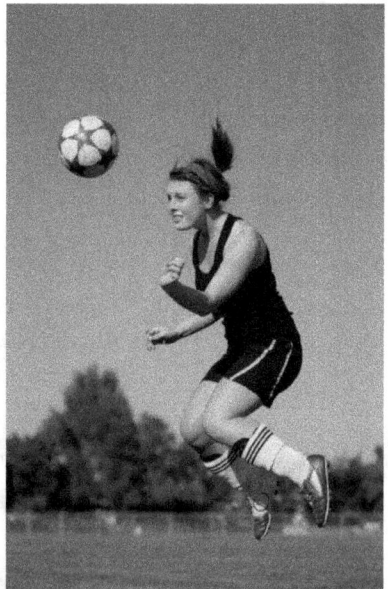

For many of us it is just not possible to incorporate exercising in our daily lives. However, there are several easy alternatives that we can adopt in order to increase our bodily activity. Simple activities like taking a walk around the office or talking the stairs instead of the elevator can improve one's level of fitness significantly.

We can also take up moderate intensity activities. These are activities that make you breathe harder or feel warmer than usual.

It is estimated that adults should do at least 150 minutes of such activities every week to stay active. One way to achieve this target is by doing 30 minutes of activity five days a week. Fit it in where you can, such as by walking or cycling to work.

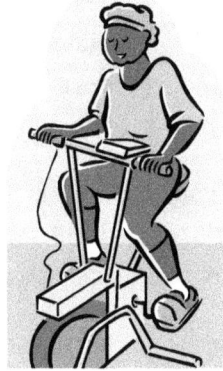

Some other types of activities that are also particularly useful are:

- ▶ **Aerobic activities:** Such activities can make you breathe harder and faster and may be moderate or vigorous in their intensity. Some aerobic activities include swimming or cycling.
  Doing aerobic exercises can give you many benefits. Perhaps the most important benefit for your life can be the reduction of your weight. Moreover, it can protect you from various diseases, such as depression, cancer and high cholesterol level.
- ▶ **Muscle-strengthening activities:** Such activities make your muscles stronger. In order to strengthen your muscles and lose weight, try weight lifting and push-

ups. While doing these activities, it is important that you utilise all the parts of your body.

▶ **Bone-strengthening activities:** Another category of activities is Bone-strengthening activities. As the name suggests, these activities strengthen your bones. These activities include jumping and hopping. These activities produce a force on the bones that promotes bone growth and strength.

If you want to look slim, then you should not just plan on reducing weight. You should, however, carefully track your progress of losing weight.

Once you start working on your body you should track your progress with a fitness and/or diet journal. Use it to note what you eat and when you ate it. This will help you keep track of your habits and help you change them for the better.

In addition to keeping your body fit you should also eat healthy food. Eating healthy food includes eating vegetables and fruits, and overlooking saturated fats and bad sugars. Change your unhealthy habits and work towards achieving a healthier lifestyle.

It may not be easy to keep yourself motivated to achieve your goals, so don't hesitate to ask a friend for help, someone who would be willing to join you and motivate you.

But the most important thing is to give yourself a reality check and ensure that you set realistic goals for yourself.

Take it slow, one thing at a time. Do not exhaust yourself from exercises. Go easy on yourself and gradually increase your exercise regime.

To conclude, by following these exercises, you should be able to keep yourself active throughout the day. Being active will not only help protect you from various diseases, it can help you reduce your bellies. Hence, if you want to look like those beautiful celebrities out there, start a healthy and active lifestyle.

Appendix I

Sample Meal Plans/Recipes

Breakfast

> 1. Buttermilk oatcakes with raspberry compote.

Nutrition facts per serving:

- ▶ 303 calories
- ▶ 5 grams fat
- ▶ 55 grams carbohydrates
- ▶ 12 grams proteins
- ▶ 9 grams fiber

Recipe:

Oatcakes:

- ▶ For oatcakes, you need to whisk 2 cups buttermilk and 1 large egg in a bowl.
- ▶ In a separate bowl, add 1 ½ cups rolled oats, ½ cup whole-wheat flour, 1 teaspoon baking soda, ½ teaspoon cinnamon, and ¼ teaspoon salt.
- ▶ Add a small quantity of water in the dry mixture to make it wet.
- ▶ Leave the batter for around 15 minutes.

Compote:

- ▶ For compote, heat 2 cups fresh raspberries, 2 tablespoons maple syrup, and 1 teaspoon of cinnamon in a saucepan.

- Cook the ingredients for around five minutes, after which switch off the heat and cover up the saucepan.
- Spray a griddle with cooking spray and use ¼ cup batter per oatcake. Cook the oatcakes until they turn brown.

The oatcake and compote is ready to serve.

2. Blueberry oat pancakes with maple yogurt

Nutrition facts per serving:

- 410 calories
- 12 grams fat
- 50 grams carbohydrates
- 26 grams proteins
- 6 grams fiber

Recipe:

- Blend 1 cup rolled oats and 1 teaspoon vanilla extract in a blender.
- When the mixture gets smooth add 1 cup blueberries in it.
- Heat a large skillet and spray with cooking spray.
- Use 2 tablespoons of batter per pancake.
- Cook the pancake until you see bubbles on the top. Flip and cook until the pancakes turn golden.
- Serve your pancakes with ¾ cup yogurt and 1 tablespoon maple syrup.

3. Banana and almond butter toast

Nutrition facts per serving:

- 280 calories
- 11 grams fat
- Monounsaturated fat 7 grams
- 6 grams proteins
- 44 grams carbohydrates
- 250 milligrams sodium

It is a quick recipe which should fill you up with all the essential nutrients you need at breakfast. It is especially convenient for all those who have to rush in the morning. It will take around 5 minutes for you to make this recipe so there is no need to skip your breakfast because of being in a hurry.

Recipe:

- For this recipe, you need to spread 1 tablespoon almond butter on toast.
- Slice 1 large banana.
- Spread the slices on the almond butter toast and enjoy this delicious breakfast.

    4.   Lemon raspberry muffins

Nutrition facts per serving:

- 185 calories
- 7 grams fat
- Monounsaturated fat 4 grams
- 4 grams proteins
- 27 grams carbohydrates
- 245 milligrams sodium

Recipe:

- Spray a 12 muffin pan with cooking spray.

- Put ½ cup sugar and 1 chopped lemon zest in a food processor. Blend until finely chopped.
- Add 1 cup non-fat buttermilk, 1/3 cup canola oil, 1 egg, and 1 teaspoon vanilla extract in the mixture.
- Blend all the above ingredients until a smooth mixture is created.
- In a separate bowl, add 1 cup all-purpose flour, 1 cup whole wheat flour, 2 teaspoons baking powder, 1 teaspoon baking soda, and ¼ teaspoon salt.
- Add the mixture created in the blender to the mixture above.
- Add 1 ½ cup raspberries to the mixture.
- Put the mixture in the muffin pan and bake the muffins for around 20 minutes.
- Take the muffins out when you see them turning golden.
- Allow them to cool and enjoy your healthy lemon raspberry muffins.

5.   Cinnamon spiked granola

Nutrition facts per serving:

- 267 calories
- 16 grams fat
- Monounsaturated fat 7 grams
- 7 grams proteins
- 28 grams carbohydrates
- 60 milligrams sodium

Recipe:

- ► Since seeds and nuts are important for your weight loss regime, here we have a breakfast consisting of both.
- ► Preheat your oven to 325°F.
- ► In a bowl, add 1 cup chopped almonds, 1 cup chopped walnuts, and 1 cup raw, unsalted pepitas (pumpkin seeds).
- ► Blend ½ cup maple syrup, 6 tablespoons canola oil, ¼ cup honey, 1 teaspoon ground cinnamon, 1 teaspoon vanilla extract, and ½ teaspoon salt in a bowl.
- ► Pour out the mixture in a pan and bake it for around an hour.
- ► While baking, stir the mixture every 15 minutes.
- ► Your granola is now ready. Allow the mixture to cool, then enjoy this yummy breakfast.

Lunch

1. *Grilled fish burger*

Nutrition facts per serving:

- 406 calories
- 8 grams fat
- Saturated fat 2.6 grams
- 50 grams proteins
- 33 grams carbohydrates
- 922 milligrams sodium

Recipe:

- Heat a griddle pan on medium heat.
- Spray 150 grams of white fish with cooking spray.
- Use salt and pepper to season your fish.
- Gently cook your fish for around 4-5 minutes.
- Gently toast the inside of a bun.
- Add 3 slices of tomato and some lettuce to the bun.
- When your fish is cooked dress your bun with the fish.
- For variety you can enjoy your fish burger with some tomato sauce as well.

2. *Pumpkin and chickpea burger (Veggie burger)*

Nutrition facts per serving:

- 401 calories
- 9 grams fat
- Saturated fat 1.6 grams
- 17 grams proteins

- ► 56 grams carbohydrates
- ► 826 milligrams sodium

Recipe:

- ► In a preheated oven (325°F), bake 200 grams of cubed pumpkin for about 20 minutes.
- ► In a blender, add 1 can of chickpeas, 1 teaspoon cumin, 1 teaspoon grounded coriander, 1 teaspoon of onion powder, 1 teaspoon of Dijon mustard, 1 teaspoon smoked paprika, ½ lemon zest, 2 cloves of garlic, salt and pepper, and some Worcestershire sauce.
- ► Blend all the above ingredients and pour the mixture out in a separate bowl.
- ► Add 2 shredded slices of bread in the mixture.
- ► Form a pattie out of the mixture and cook it until it turns golden and crispy.
- ► Add tomatoes, lettuce, yogurt, and chili sauce on your rolls. Fill your rolls with the pattie, and enjoy a tasty lunch.

   3. Rice vermicelli with prawns

Nutrition facts per serving:

- ► 303 calories
- ► 8 grams fat
- ► Saturated fat 1.3 grams
- ► 21 grams proteins
- ► 32 grams carbohydrates
- ► 1400 milligrams sodium

Recipe:

► Soak 120 grams of vermicelli noodles in boiling water for around 4 minutes.

► Pour the water out and allow the noodles to cool.

► In the meantime fry ½ sliced onions and ½ red sliced capsicums (peppers).

► Add 150 grams of prawns in the pan and stir them for a few minutes.

► Add 2 cloves of crushed garlic and ½ teaspoon of red chili paste.

► Add the fried vegetables in the pan and mix well.

► Mix the noodles in the pan as well. Add 1-2 teaspoons of sauces in the pan and cook for a few minutes.

► Tasty rice vermicelli with prawns ready to serve.

4. *Roasted capsicum (pepper) stuffed with quinoa (whole grain: pronounced KEEN-wah)*

Nutrition facts per serving:

► 126 calories
► 4 grams fat
► Saturated fat 1.6 grams
► 7.4 grams proteins
► 13 grams carbohydrates
► 57 milligrams sodium

Recipe:

► Preheat your oven to 350F.
► Take ½ cup quinoa and cook it with 1 cup water. Cook on medium-low heat 10 to 15 minutes or until all liquid is absorbed.

- Allow the quinoa to cool.
- Cut 2-3 large capsicums in half. Remove their seeds.
- Take 1 diced tomato, 1 chopped celery stick, 1 sliced spring onion, 1 clove of garlic, some oregano, 1 tablespoon chopped parsley, ½ cup ricotta, and 4 chopped button mushrooms.
- Mix all these ingredients in a bowl and add the quinoa.
- Fill the capsicums with this mixture.
- Bake your capsicums for around 40 minutes.
- Your vegetarian lunch is ready to serve.

5. Frittata

Nutrition facts per serving:

- 322 calories
- 16 grams fat
- Saturated fat 5.6 grams
- 35 grams proteins
- 9 grams carbohydrates
- 611 milligrams sodium

Recipe:

- Preheat your oven to 350F.
- Fry ¼ sliced onions and ¼ chorizo sausages in a non-stick pan for around 5 minutes.
- Make sure that the onions have softened.
- In a bowl mix together 8 eggs, 1/3 cup low fat milk, some garlic powder, some dried oregano, 1 teaspoon of wholegrain mustard.
- Also add some salt and pepper for taste to the mixture.

- ▶ In a baking tray make a layer of the onion mixture first. Add some tomatoes in the middle layer.
- ▶ Add the egg mixture on top of the tomatoes. Make sure all the layers are evenly spread.
- ▶ Your dish will be ready after baking it for around 40 minutes.

Dinner

1. *Creamy chicken and broccoli*

Nutrition facts per serving:

- ▶ 425 calories
- ▶ 9 grams fat
- ▶ Saturated fat 4 grams
- ▶ 50 grams proteins
- ▶ 32 grams carbohydrates
- ▶ 446 milligrams sodium

Recipe:

- ▶ Heat 4 medium sized potatoes in a microwave oven for around 10 minutes.
- ▶ Preheat your oven to 350F.
- ▶ Fry ½ sliced onions and chorizo in a fry pan for around 5 minutes. After adding 1 head of cut up broccoli to the pan, fry for further 4 minutes.
- ▶ In a bowl and add 1 can of evaporated milk, 2 teaspoons of regular mustard, 2 teaspoons of Dijon mustard, 1 clove garlic, and some salt and pepper.
- ▶ Add the mixture to 1 BBQ chicken.
- ▶ Place sliced potatoes on top.
- ▶ Add some cheese on top. Bake for around 30 minutes.

2. *Grilled fish with creamy lemon and basil sauce*

Nutrition facts per serving:

- ▶ 557 calories

- 16 grams fat
- Saturated fat 5.2 grams
- 60 grams proteins
- 37 grams carbohydrates
- 580 milligrams sodium

Recipe:

- Preheat your oven up to 400F.
- Put 12 cherry tomatoes and 3 large unpeeled garlic cloves in a baking tray.
- Sprinkle a few drops of olive oil and allow the two items to bake for around 30 minutes.
- While the cherry tomatoes are being baked, blend 1 can white beans, 1 crushed garlic clove, sour cream, and 1 tablespoon lemon. Also sprinkle some salt and pepper for seasoning.
- You can also alter the amount of lemon and garlic added in the blender according to your taste.
- Cook 2 fish fillets of 150 grams in a fry pan, cooking both sides.
- After cooking for a few minutes bake the fish for around 20 minutes.
- Take half of the tomatoes you baked earlier. Blend them with 12 basil leaves, the juice of 1 lemon, and 1 cup light evaporated milk.
- Add salt and pepper for taste in the blender.
- Once the mixture is smooth pour it out in a pan and warm it on low heat.
- Take 1 teaspoon corn flour and add it to 2 tablespoons of cold water.

► Add this corn flour in the warm mixture above. Keep on stirring the mixture until it becomes thick in consistency.

► Your sauce is now ready. Serve this sauce and the remaining half cherry tomatoes with the freshly baked fish.

3. Tuna and broccoli stir fry

Nutrition facts per serving:

► 370 calories
► 16 grams fat
► Saturated fat 2.6 grams
► 42 grams proteins
► 12 grams carbohydrates
► 952 milligrams sodium

Recipe:

► Using 2 tablespoon olive oil, fry ½ sliced onions, and ¼ sliced capsicums for around 5 minutes.

► Steam the broccoli for a few minutes by placing 2 cups broccoli with ¼ cup water in a pan.

► Let all the water evaporate and then add chunks of 1 large tuna steak to the pan.

► Using one drop of olive oil, mix the tuna chunks and the vegetables.

► To prepare the sauce use 2 tablespoons of soy sauce, 1 tablespoon of crushed garlic, 1 tablespoon of crushed ginger, and 1 tablespoon of rice wine vinegar.

► Add this sauce to the tuna. Keep on stirring until the sauce is properly mixed and cooked.

- Your dish is now ready to serve. You can also add some sesame seeds for garnishing.

4. *Spanish chicken and rice*

Nutrition facts per serving:

- 598 calories
- 26 grams fat
- Saturated fat 7.4 grams
- 55 grams proteins
- 28 grams carbohydrates
- 374 milligrams sodium

Recipe:

- Preheat your oven up to 375F.
- For a few minutes fry ½ sliced onion. Once it is done, fry ½ chorizos.
- In the onion and chorizo mixture, add 1 teaspoon smoked paprika, ½ teaspoon sweet paprika, some oregano, and 3 crushed garlic cloves.
- After you cook the above ingredients for 2 minutes add ¾ cup rice, 1 ½ cups of chicken stock, 1 can of butter beans, and paprika. Cook for a few minutes and then take it off the stove.
- Place the rice mixture in a baking dish and squeeze 2 tablespoons lemon juice on the top. Place it in the oven after covering it tightly with foil.
- Take chunks of 1 large chicken breast and fry it in the oil. Allow the chicken to turn brown, around 5 minutes.
- Add 2 garlic cloves on the top and cook for another minute.

- ▶ When the rice has been cooked properly in the oven, take it out and add ½ cup peas, and 1 large chopped tomato. Add your chicken and garlic mixture to the rice, and cook it for another 20 minutes by covering it tightly with the foil.
- ▶ Your Spanish chicken and rice is now ready to eat.

5. *Vegetarian fried rice*

Nutrition facts per serving:

- ▶ 358 calories
- ▶ 7.6 grams fat
- ▶ Saturated fat 1.9 grams
- ▶ 12 grams proteins
- ▶ 56 grams carbohydrates
- ▶ 1390 milligrams sodium

Recipe:

- ▶ Fry 1 medium onion under low heat for around 2 minutes.
- ▶ Sauté 1 chopped carrot, 1 chopped celery stick, ½ chopped zucchini; 2 tablespoons crushed ginger and ½ chopped red capsicum.
- ▶ Sauté the above ingredients for 5 minutes then add 3 tablespoons of soy sauce.
- ▶ Beat 2 eggs with 2 tablespoons of low fat milk and add it to the vegetable mixture above.
- ▶ After adding the eggs, place ½ can corn and 8 sliced mushrooms in the vegetable mixture.
- ▶ Make sure to continue stirring as you add new ingredients.

- ► Cook 3 cups of rice and mix them with the vegetables.
- ► Add soy sauce and oyster sauce on top of the rice.
- ► Your dish is now ready to serve.

Snacks

1. *Potato snack*

Nutrition facts per serving:

- ► 253 calories
- ► 5.7 grams fat
- ► Saturated fat 0.6 grams
- ► 6.3 grams proteins
- ► 40 grams carbohydrates
- ► 489 milligrams sodium

Recipe:

- ► Preheat your oven to 400F.
- ► Slice 600 grams of baby potatoes.
- ► Coat them with a few drops of olive oil.
- ► Place the potatoes in a baking tray and bake them for around 15 minutes.
- ► After the initial 15 minutes add dried rosemary leaves on top of the potatoes.
- ► Put them back into the oven for 5 more minutes.
- ► Take them out of the oven once they are properly baked and add salt according to your taste.
- ► Your healthy potato snack is now ready to eat.

2. *Banana, apple and oat cookies*

Nutrition facts per serving:

- ► 105 calories
- ► 5 grams fat
- ► Saturated fat 0.5 grams

- 2 grams proteins
- 12 grams carbohydrates
- 16 milligrams sodium

Recipe:

- Preheat your oven up to 375F.
- Mix 1 cup rolled oats, ¾ cup almond meal, 1 teaspoon cinnamon, and ½ teaspoon baking powder in a bowl.
- Beat one egg lightly and add half of it to the ingredients above.
- To the remaining egg add 2 tablespoons of olive oil and 2 tablespoons of golden syrup, and add this to the oats and almond mixture.
- Mash 2 bananas with a fork and add to the mixture above.
- Also add 1 cubed apple.
- Mix all the ingredients well and make cookies out of the mixture.
- Put these cookies in the oven and allow them to cook for 20 minutes.
- Before eating all of the cookies, note that this recipe will make 16 servings.

   3.   *Gluten free banana cake*

Nutrition facts per serving:

- 220 calories
- 4.9 grams fat
- Saturated fat 0.8 grams
- 10 grams proteins
- 36 grams carbohydrates

► 258 milligrams sodium

Recipe:

► Preheat your oven up to 350F.
► Add 1 cup rice flour, 1 teaspoon cinnamon, ½ cup almond meal, 1 teaspoon baking powder, and ½ cup sugar in a large bowl.
► In this mixture add 2 tablespoons of melted margarine.
► While stirring, add 1 egg, ½ cup low fat yogurt, and 1 teaspoon vanilla essence.
► Place ½ cup almond milk in a microwave for around 40 seconds. When the almond milk is heated up, add 1 teaspoon of baking soda.
► Add this almond milk mixture into the rice flour mixture.
► Mix them well and then add 3 mashed bananas.
► Add 2 egg whites to the mixture. Make sure to mix everything well after you add half of the egg whites.
► Place the mixture in the oven for 40 minutes and enjoy this healthy snack.

4. *Apple and cinnamon muffins*

Nutrition facts per serving:

► 207 calories
► 4 grams fat
► Saturated fat 1.2 grams
► 5.2 grams proteins
► 36 grams carbohydrates
► 155 milligrams sodium

Recipe:

- ▶ Preheat your oven up to 350F.
- ▶ Cook 2 chopped apples along with 1 tablespoon water and some cinnamon for around 10 minutes.
- ▶ In a bowl place 2 tablespoons of light margarine and ½ cup castor sugar. Beat the two ingredients.
- ▶ Add 1 teaspoon of vanilla essence and beat for a further 1 minute.
- ▶ To this mixture add 2 eggs and ½ cup low fat yogurt.
- ▶ Mix 1 cup flour with 1 teaspoon of baking powder.
- ▶ Add this flour mixture to the apple and egg mixture.
- ▶ Make sure you carefully mix all the ingredients while adding. Fill the muffin pans.
- ▶ Let the muffins bake for 20 minutes.
- ▶ A healthy snack is now ready to eat.
- ▶ Before you eat all of the muffins, note that this recipe will create 8 servings.

5. *Peach and fig baby cakes*

Nutrition facts per serving:

- ▶ 148 calories
- ▶ 2.7 grams fat
- ▶ Saturated fat 0.9 grams
- ▶ 4.2 grams proteins
- ▶ 26 grams carbohydrates
- ▶ 114 milligrams sodium

Recipe:

- ▶ Preheat your oven up to 350F.
- ▶ Beat 3 tablespoons of margarine and 1/3 cup of castor sugar for 5 minutes. Add ½ grated lemon rind and 1

teaspoon of vanilla essence and beat for 1 more minute.

▶ While beating at a slow speed add 2 eggs, 2 teaspoons of low fat yogurt and 1/3 cup of low fat milk.

▶ Mix 1 cup plain flour with 1 teaspoon of baking powder, and add it to the margarine and egg mixture above.

▶ Add 8 chopped peaches and 6 dried figs to the mixture. Carefully mix all the ingredients.

▶ Place this mixture in a pan and allow it to bake for 20 minutes.

▶ Before consuming all of the healthy muffins, note that this recipe will create 10 servings. If you eat 2 muffins, you will get double the nutrition mentioned above.

Appendix II

Frequently Asked Questions

Q. If I have a family history of being overweight, does that mean I will never be able to lose weight?

This is a serious concern of many people who are trying to lose weight. Most people are overweight because they consume more calories than they burn off daily. Unfortunately, a person's tendency to gain weight does increase if he or she has a family history of being overweight.

You may have noticed a family where almost everyone has gained weight. In such a family, it is a common misconception that they will never be able to lose weight, just because of their genes.

They believe that they will always remain obese, no matter how much they try. As a result, often they do not try losing weight, and consequently do in fact gain additional weight, putting themselves at a higher risk of having additional problems because of their weight.

GOOD NEWS! It has been proven by research that you can lose weight even if you have a genetic inheritance of being overweight. You can burn off the extra fat and calories by exercising and reducing your calorie intake.

Start walking and running, watch your calories, and soon you should see a difference in your body weight, despite the fact that you have 'overweight' genes.

Q. Why have I started gaining weight, despite the fact that I am exercising regularly?

You may face this problem, especially if you have recently started exercising. Many people gain weight when they start their exercise regime. Your exercise regime is not to be blamed though. There can be many factors which can lead you to gain weight.

Inappropriate diet can be one of the reasons for weight gain while exercising. It is often seen that when you start exercising, your appetite increases. You may crave for more food. This may result in you cheating on yourself, and you may consume a few extra calories. This can then become the reason for weight gain.

To avoid this problem, note the responses of your body when you feel hungry. Normally the hunger feeling comes when you feel both tired and weak. If you do not feel tired, and still feel hungry, your body is probably playing tricks on you. This is probably a sign that you are just craving more food.

To avoid eating extra food, keep tempting foods out of your reach.

Also, you can divert your mind for 20 minutes if your body craves for extra food. Research has shown that waiting for 20 minutes can help to reduce the cravings. Try drinking a glass of water and waiting to see if the cravings go away.

By following these tips you can avoid gaining more weight during your weight loss regime.

Q. I think I am reducing my carbohydrate intake too much. What should I do?

A common mistake made by people starting a new weight-loss program is to reduce their carbohydrate intake to a dangerously low level. You should never do this. Since carbohydrates are essential for your wellbeing, you should not completely eliminate them from your diet.

You should just reduce their quantity, ensuring that you consume the daily recommended levels. To avoid problems for your body you should also consume fruits and vegetables to fill you up with the lost energy.

Also, ensure that you are consuming enough fiber. This is because fiber is a good source of energy for your body.

If you eat vegetables, fruits and fibers, and do not eliminate carbohydrates from your diet, you should be able to continue with your weight loss regime.

Q. Will eating late at night increase my weight?

Everyone does not work a standard 9-5 schedule. Lots of people working evening and late shifts. It is common for these people to have their dinners at a time when other people are sleeping. If you are one of these 'late-nighters', then do not fear, read on.

The timing of when you eat is not the key factor. It is the quantity. If you consume the recommended level of calories, combined with regular exercise, you should be fine.

Remember that the essential nutrients are important to avoid weight gain.

However, if you buy junk food and eat it at night, there are very high chances that this can cause you to gain weight.

As long as you can manage to take in less calories and burn more of them, you should not gain weight even if you eat late at night.

Q. Will it make a difference if I replace table salt with sea salt?

High consumption of salt can be dangerous for your health. It can lead you to gain weight. This is because salt contains a high quantity of sodium, which has the ability to retain water in your body.

Both sea salt and table salt are made up of sodium and chlorine. Since they both contain almost equal quantities of sodium, it will not make a big difference if you replace one with another.

Either can lead you to gain weight if used to excess.

Sea salt is preferred by many people because it contains extra minerals. However, these extra minerals are in such a small quantity that they normally do not increase your daily mineral intake.

Therefore, there is little difference between the two salts.

Salts in general should be reduced by a person who wants to reduce his or her weight. Instead of replacing one source of sodium with another source, one could consider using potassium salts.

Q. Will I burn more fat if I exercise with an empty stomach?

It is a common belief that exercising with an empty stomach fastens the fat burning process. It is a common practice of many people to exercise just after they get up.

The reason why many people do this is because when you are in a state of fasting, your blood sugar levels are low. It is the reduced quantity of sugar levels in the blood which helps fasten the process of fat burning.

When you exercise with an empty stomach, you use more fat for fuel, but this does not mean that the fat is actually being burnt away.

When you exercise with an empty stomach you may not be able to exercise for long. This is because your body will not have enough energy to continue the exercises.

If you exercise with an empty stomach you may not be able to burn more fat. It is therefore advisable that you eat something before you exercise. In this way your body will have more energy to carry on with the exercises, and you will be able to burn more fat overall.

A glass of juice or a piece of fruit is enough energy to get you going before exercise.

Q. Should I rely on the calorie counter on the gym exercise machines?

You will often find exercise machines in the gym which will tell you the amount of calories you will burn while exercising. These machines use a formula to figure out the number of calories being burnt off. However, these formulas are not always reliable. One should not rely just on the calorie counter provided by the exercise machines in the gym.

Some of the measures used to calculate the calories are inaccurate. They miss out several factors such as the percentage of fat in your body.

Having a high percentage of fat is one thing, while having a high muscle mass is another thing. A person having a high muscle mass will burn more calories as compared to the person having a higher percentage of fat.

Also, if you have recently started exercising, you will burn more calories. On the other hand, if a person has been exercising for a long time, he or she is less likely to burn more calories.

The calorie count on the machines will not take these factors into account, and will thus be an inaccurate measure.

Some machines have the tendency to overestimate the number of calories by 10-15%.

Instead of relying on these numbers, one should rely on other measures to count the number of calories burnt while exercising. There are a number of good tools available on the web. Do a Google search and you will find many, from the simple and basic, to the more thorough and reliable.

Q. Can I take a day or two off from my weight loss diet on weekends?

Many people take one or two days off from their diets. They usually fulfill their wishes of eating their favourite high calorie foods once or twice on weekends. This is a dangerous practice to follow. This is because it can sometimes ruin your chances of losing weight.

Your diet on weekends is important for your weight loss regime. With a lot of leisure time available on weekends there can be a tendency to consume more food. On the hand, your busy schedule on weekdays may not allow you to concentrate on eating out for pleasure.

If you follow a diet in which you take weekends off, make sure you eat within the limits defined. Watch your calorie intake. You should also exercise and burn off the calories gained. If you do not do so, you may decrease the effectiveness of the diet which you have followed for the whole week.

Q. I am following my friend's weight loss strategy. Why am I not losing weight?

Do you have a friend who has successfully lost weight? Seeing him or her getting back into shape, you may be tempted to follow your friend's strategy. You should, however, be careful if you do this.

Every person has different needs. Your bodily needs may be different from the needs of your friend. He or she may have different strategies to lose weight which may not necessarily work for you.

For example, your friend may not need a tough exercise regime to burn his or her fat. Your body, on the other hand, may contain more fat than your friend. The amount of exercise needed by you may be more than the amount needed by your friend.

In this case, if you follow in your friend's footsteps and exercise less, you may end up gaining weight instead. It is advisable to make your own weight loss schedule. See what works best for your body. Stick to that regime instead of following what regime worked best for your friend.

Q. It is difficult for me to reduce my consumption of sweets. Can I eat sweets with low calories?

Sweets can be dangerous for your weight loss regime. They can make or break your chances of getting back into shape. The sugars contained in some sweets can be dangerous for your health and may increase your weight.

It is normally advised that you reduce your intake of sweets. It is when you reduce the intake of sweets that you should be more successful in reducing your weight. However, if a sudden reduction is creating problems for you, try reducing the consumption slowly and gradually.

To gradually reduce your consumption of sweets, you can consume sweets with fewer calories. To do this, make sure you read the labels on the sweets before you buy them. You should buy the items which will give you less than 150 calories per serving. Examples of such sweets include sugar-free gelatin, frozen fruit juice, and fat free milk.

Eating low-calorie sweets may help initially. You should gradually reduce your consumption of sweets. If you gradually reduce your consumption, your body should adapt to the change in your diet. You should then not face problems.

It is not dangerous if you initially consume low calorie sweets, but you should slowly reduce the consumption if you want to lose weight successfully.

Q. Will it affect my weight loss regime if I skip meals to reduce my calorie intake?

Skipping meals to reduce your weight is a complete no-no. Skipping meals is a very dangerous practice to follow. If you want to effectively reduce your weight, then you should forget about skipping meals.

You may get upset and disappointed when you see your bloated body. In an attempt to quickly lose weight, many people skip meals. However, your chances of consuming more calories may increase if you plan on skipping meals.

If you starve yourself, you may feel a lot hungrier. If this happens, you may end up eating more than is required by your body. Your weight may increase and your strategy of starving may fail.

Therefore, it is strongly advised that you do not skip meals. Do consume food regularly. The consumption, however, should be in a limited amount. It should also be within the daily recommended levels.

Q. Should I go for the magic diets and reduce weight within a few days?

Just like skipping meals, magic diets too are strictly not advisable. These magic diets can be harmful for your body and weight in the long run.

These products may look very tempting at first sight. They promise to get you back in shape within a few days or a few weeks. No matter how much you want to lose weight fast, you should not use such products.

These products may reduce your weight quickly, but the chances of relapse will probably increase. There may be higher chances of you gaining weight again. Also, some of these products may be damaging for your health.

Therefore, stick to a proper weight loss regime, no matter how hard and slow it seems to be. These weight loss regimes can successfully reduce your weight, and without the associated risk that potential come with the magic diets.

Q. If I consume 100 calories of two different foods, will I gain the same amount of weight?

It is generally true that all calories are created equal. This means that if you eat 100 calories of chocolate and 100 calories of a fruit, you will gain equal amounts of weight from these two foods.

However, there are certain foods which are more satiating then others. As an example, you normally feel fuller if you consume 100 calories of bananas, as compared to 100 calories of chicken. Also, 100 calories of bananas may give you more nutrients than 100 calories of chicken.

Thus, although foods with equal calories may cause equal amount of weight gain, their impact on your weight loss regime may be different. You should, therefore, choose your foods wisely.

Q. How often should I check my weight?

You may hear various opinions on this issue. Some people may advise you to weigh yourself regularly, while others may suggest you to wait till the weekend.

The frequency of checking your weight should depend on your own schedule and bodily requirements. For example, if you are diabetic or a person with heart problems, then it may be advisable for you to monitor your weight daily.

Whatever schedule you choose, if possible, weight yourself at roughly the same time of the day. That helps give a better indication of your weight.

Body weight can change throughout the day, depending on intake of food, exercise and just normal body functions. If you weight yourself today after dinner and compare it to your weight from yesterday just after waking up, it could be quite different.

Q. What should I do to maintain my weight once I reduce it?

If you have been successful in reducing your weight, then you should not abruptly leave your diet and exercise regimes. If you do so, there are chances that the lost pounds may come back.

To stay in shape, you should continue with moderate activities. Research has shown that people, who have continued their exercises even after losing weight, have successfully maintained their weight.

You should also not leave your diet. Continue with the low calorie diet and a proper exercise regime to keep the lost pounds at bay.

Dear Reader,

We hope you enjoyed and benefited from this publication.

Make sure you don't miss out on exciting and practical information from our Health, Fitness & Dieting blog. Join our Preferred Customer list and stay in touch with Durango's Email Tips & Tricks for Weight Loss the healthy and natural way. You will get advance emails on:

1. New diet plans
2. Flash news
3. Weight loss developments
4. Plus advance notice of upcoming Special Reports and new books

Click here to sign up now:
http://www.durangopublishing.com/tipstricks/

Cheers,

Sam Martin

Marketing Manager

Other Titles By Durango Publishing Corp.®

Health, Fitness & Dieting Series
How To Supercharge YOUR Metabolism For Faster
Weight Loss

Mike Shant Mystery Series
Policy Terminated
The Conversion
Lose Weight – While We Scam
"W.I.M.P.S."

Make Money Enjoyably Series
Make To Make Big Money As An Information Publisher
How To Make Big Money Writing

Betting and WINNING Horse Races Series
Horse Racing: Gambling to Win
Vegas Pro's Best Racing Angles
Horse Racing – 3 Year Olds

Fiction
The Day B.C. Quit Canada
The God Franchise

Available at:
www.DurangoPublishing.com
&
http://goo.gl/qeUWzk

About the Authors

Wendell & Clarissa Swinton

Teamed up for their first Durango Publishing book, "YOUR 'Lose Weight FAST the Natural & Healthy-Way DIET', a simple healthy weight loss diet so YOU can live a better, happier, more enjoyable life!", this husband and wife team were richly equipped for researching and writing what may become the accepted reference in the booming Healthy Diet field.

Wendell Swinton did graduate work in nutrition and health. Following that he acted as an assistant editor on the Laurencom Publications newsletter, "Live Healthy 24/7". His responsibilities included all major projects for the monthly newsletter. He also initiated information products in areas of his special interest, including healthy weight loss and careful eating habits.

"Live Healthy 24/7"™ was later purchased by Durango Publishing Corp., and was Wendell's introduction to this rapidly growing publisher of niche specialty books and information products.

By the time of the newsletter sale Wendell had become editor-in-chief, and he was responsible for devising and assigning every major research and publishing project initiated by the newsletter. Readership was worldwide, and gave Wendell a solid understanding of how important personal health was to everyone everywhere.

Clarissa Swinton graduated with a BSc in Health Sciences, and immediately began freelance researching and writing in her chosen field. One of her first assignments was on "Personal health habits of coeds", assigned by an asst. editor of the popular newsletter "Live Healthy 24/7".

She completed the assignment and received a glowing letter of appreciation "for a thoroughly researched and written article" by that asst. editor, Wendell Swinton, who in the fullness of time became her husband. "But not before we had worked together on a number of projects, and I realized that he was as serious about the healthy diet and nutrition field as I was," Clarissa laughed.

Now, with publication of "YOUR 'Lose Weight FAST the Natural & Healthy-Way DIET', a simple healthy weight loss diet so YOU can live a better, happier, more enjoyable life!" Wendell and Clarissa have fulfilled a long standing desire to work together.

Both Wendell and Clarissa would love feedback from you, especially if you have an idea or suggestion for a future book or course in Durango's expanding "Live Healthy 24/7"® line of books and information products. Contact them directly at:

Wendell@DurangoPublishing.com

Clarissa@DurangoPublishing.com

And if you would like advance information on the wonderful online courses already in the research stage, simply send an email to editor@durangopublishing.com and mention "Course Information" in the subject line.

Dear Reader,

Thank you so much for reading our book. We hope you really liked it, and found it helpful in setting and following your healthy nutrition and weight-loss goals.

As you probably know, many people look at the reviews on Amazon before they decide to purchase a book.

If you liked the book, could you please take a minute to leave a 4 or 5 star review with your feedback?

You can do that right here.

Amazon: http://www.amazon.com/YOUR-Lose-Weight-Natural-Healthy-Way-ebook/dp/B00J8ZP0JO

60 seconds is all we are asking for, and it would mean the world to us. Your friendly help will certainly help us in further research & writing.

Thank you so much, and here's to weight loss the healthy and natural way.

Wendell & Clarissa Swinton